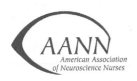

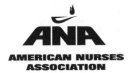

Neuroscience Nursing

Scope AND Standards OF PRACTICE

2ND EDITION

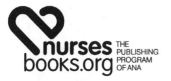

nurses THE PUBLISHING PROGRAM books.org OF ANA

American Nurses Association
Silver Spring, Maryland
2013

American Nurses Association
8515 Georgia Avenue, Suite 400
Silver Spring, MD 20910-3492
1-800-274-4ANA
http://www.NursingWorld.org

Published by Nursesbooks.org
The Publishing Program of ANA
http://www.Nursesbooks.org/

The American Association of Neuroscience Nurses (AANN) and the American Nurses Association (ANA) are national professional associations. This joint AANN and ANA publication—*Neuroscience Nursing: Scope and Standards of Practice, 2nd Edition*—reflects the thinking of the practice specialty of holistic nursing on various issues and should be reviewed in conjunction with state board of nursing policies and practices. State law, rules, and regulations govern the practice of nursing, while *Neuroscience Nursing: Scope and Standards of Practice, 2nd Edition,* guides nurses in the application of their professional skills and responsibilities.

The American Association of Neuroscience Nurses (AANN) is committed to working for the highest standard of care for neuroscience patients by advancing the science and practice of neuroscience nursing. Founded in 1968, the AANN accomplishes this through continuing education, information dissemination, standard setting, and advocacy on behalf of neuroscience patients, families, and nurses. AANN develops and supports nurses in providing excellence in care and promotes the neuroscience nursing specialty. As the leading authority in neuroscience nursing, AANN inspires passion in nurses and creates the future for the specialty.

The American Nurses Association (ANA) is the only full-service professional organization representing the interests of the nation's 3.1 million registered nurses through its constituent/state nurses associations and its organizational affiliates. The ANA advances the nursing profession by fostering high standards of nursing practice, promoting the rights of nurses in the workplace, projecting a positive and realistic view of nursing, and by lobbying the Congress and regulatory agencies on health care issues affecting nurses and the public.

Library of Congress Cataloging-in-Publication available on request.

ISBN-13: 978-1-55810-503-4   SAN: 851-3481   03/2013

First printing: March 2013

Contents

Contributors

Neuroscience Nursing Standards Workforce 2012–13

Chris Stewart-Amidei, RN, PhD, CNRN, FAAN, Task Force Chairperson
Susan Bell, RN, MS, CNRN, CNP
Ambre Pownall, RN, MSN
Laura Reese, RN, MSN, CNRN
Bridget Solomon, RN, BSN
Catherine Stephens, RN, MSN, CNRN
Misti Tuppery, RN, MSN, CNRN, CCRN, CCNS
AANN Board of Director's Liaison, Janice L. Hinkle, RN, PhD, CNRN
AANN Staff Liaison, Joan Kram, RN, MBA, FACHE

ANA Staff

Carol Bickford, PhD, RN-BC, CPHIMS – Content editor
Maureen E. Cones, Esq. – Legal counsel
Yvonne Daley Humes, MSA – Project coordinator
Eric Wurzbacher, BA – Project editor

About the American Association of Neuroscience Nurses

Founded in 1968, the American Association of Neuroscience Nurses (AANN) is committed to working for the highest standard of care for neuroscience patients by advancing the science and practice of neuroscience nursing. AANN accomplishes this through continuing education, information dissemination, standard setting, and advocacy on behalf of neuroscience patients, families, and nurses. AANN develops and supports nurses in providing excellence in

care and promotes the neuroscience nursing specialty. As the leading authority in neuroscience nursing, AANN inspires passion in nurses and creates the
future for the specialty.

About the American Nurses Association

The American Nurses Association (ANA) is the only full-service professional
organization representing the interests of the nation's 3.1 million registered
nurses through its constituent/state nurses associations and its organizational
affiliates. The ANA advances the nursing profession by fostering high standards
of nursing practice, promoting the rights of nurses in the workplace, projecting a positive and realistic view of nursing, and by lobbying the Congress and
regulatory agencies on healthcare issues affecting nurses and the public.

About Nursesbooks.org, The
Publishing Program of ANA

Nursesbooks.org publishes books on ANA core issues and programs, including
ethics, leadership, quality, specialty practice, advanced practice, and the profession's enduring legacy. Best known for the foundational documents of the
profession on nursing ethics, scope and standards of practice, and social policy,
Nursesbooks.org is the publisher for the professional, career-oriented nurse,
reaching and serving nurse educators, administrators, managers, and researchers as well as staff nurses in the course of their professional development.

Preface

Neuroscience nursing is a nursing specialty that addresses the needs and care of individuals with biological, psychological, social, and spiritual alterations as a result of nervous system dysfunction. Registered nurses and advanced practice registered nurses (APRNs) specializing in the practice of neuroscience nursing are challenged to provide care to patients and families within a complex and constantly changing healthcare environment. The roles of neuroscience registered nurses and APRNs are multifaceted and dynamic. It is crucial for neuroscience registered nurses and APRNs to be aware of the diverse statutes and regulations governing their practice and be able to perform within their defined scope of practice. This document is intended to assist the neuroscience registered nurse and APRN in developing a framework for practice.

Setting the Stage

Foundational Documents

Neuroscience Nursing: Scope and Standards of Practice describes components of competent nursing practice and professional performance in the specialized field of neuroscience nursing. This document outlines the expectations of the professional role of the neuroscience nurse, identifies the scope of practice, and presents the standards of professional nursing practice with accompanying competencies for all neuroscience nurses.

Nurses practicing neuroscience nursing in the United States have several key foundational resources to inform and guide their practice. First, tenets of an ethical framework for neuroscience nurses practicing across all roles, settings, and levels of practice are identified through *Code of Ethics for Nurses with Interpretive Statements* (ANA, 2001) and *Guide to the Code of Ethics for Nurses: Interpretation and Application* (Fowler, 2008). Another significant foundational document is *Nursing's Social Policy Statement: The Essence of the Profession* (ANA, 2010b), which conceptualizes nursing practice, describes the social context of nursing, and provides the definition of nursing. The final foundational resource is *Nursing: Scope and Standards of Practice, 2nd ed.* (ANA, 2010a). The scope and standards of neuroscience nursing practice have been developed from these documents.

Audience

Registered and advanced practice registered nurses specializing in neuroscience nursing constitute the primary audience for this professional resource. Healthcare providers and interprofessional colleagues, as well as administrators practicing in healthcare systems, agencies, and organizations, will find this a valuable reference in understanding the roles of neuroscience registered nurses and APRNs. In addition, patients, families, communities, and populations using neuroscience nursing services can use this document to better understand what constitutes the practice of neuroscience nursing and who its members are: registered nurses and APRNs specializing in neuroscience nursing. Finally, legislators, regulators, legal counsel, and the judiciary system may wish to reference this document to better understand what constitutes the practice of neuroscience nursing.

Scope of Neuroscience Nursing Practice

Definitions and Distinguishing Characteristics of Neuroscience Nursing Practice

Definitions

Nursing is defined as "the protection, promotion, and optimization of health and abilities, prevention of illness and injury, alleviation of suffering through the diagnosis and treatment of human response, and advocacy in the care of individuals, families, communities, and populations" (ANA, 2010a, p. 1; ANA, 2010b, p. 10).

Neuroscience nursing is defined as a nursing specialty that addresses the needs and care of individuals with biological, psychological, social, and spiritual alterations as a result of nervous system dysfunction (Webb, 2000). This encompasses all levels of human existence, from basic bodily functions to advanced processes of the human mind. Neuroscience nurses identify and treat human responses to actual or potential health problems related to phenomena affected by nervous system dysfunction. Phenomena addressed within the context of neuroscience nursing practice include: consciousness and cognition, communication, affiliate relationships, mobility, rest and sleep, sensation, elimination, sexuality, self-care, and integrated regulation. Potential recipients of neuroscience nursing care are individuals with nervous system dysfunction, their families and significant others, and the society in which they live.

Distinguishing Characteristics

The American Nurses Association (ANA) identifies the following essential features of nursing practice:

- A caring relationship that facilitates health and healing. In neuroscience nursing, this relationship is critically important when individuals are unable to speak for themselves due to an altered level of responsiveness.

- Attention to a range of human experiences and responses to health, disease, and illness in the physical and social environments. In neuroscience nursing, this might include assessing the home environment to which a person with quadriplegia will return.

- Integration of objective data with knowledge gained from an appreciation of the patient's or group's subjective experience. An example is planning an educational program for caregivers of persons with Alzheimer's disease based on assessment of their needs.

- Application of scientific knowledge to diagnosis and treatment through the use of judgment and critical thinking. Neuroscience nurses are adept at critically distinguishing the significance of findings from the neurologic exams they conduct.

- Advancement of professional nursing knowledge through scholarly inquiry. For example, neuroscience nurses have increased compliance with seizure medication regimens by evaluating factors that enhance compliance.

- Influence on social and public policy to promote social justice. For example, neuroscience nurses have participated in efforts to require seat belt and helmet use in order to prevent neurologic injury.

- Assurance of safe, quality, and evidence-based practice. For example, neuroscience nurses incorporate quality measures, such as swallow evaluations, into care of the patient with stroke.

(ANA, 2010a, p. 29; ANA, 2010b, p. 9)

These essential features are applied in neuroscience nursing practice to address the phenomena unique to the specialty.

Specific phenomena defined by the American Association of Neuroscience Nurses (AANN) that comprise the unique domain of neuroscience nursing include:

- *Consciousness and cognition*—The awareness of and interaction with the surrounding environment as well as the higher thought processes; alterations include problems such as coma, memory impairment, and seizures.

- *Communication*—The language interaction with others; alterations include language impairments secondary to the aphasias or dysarthria.

- *Affiliate relationships*—The ability to form and maintain social support relationships; alterations include social isolation and role changes secondary to nervous system disease.

- *Mobility*—The ability to move freely within the environment; alterations include various forms of paralysis.

- *Rest and sleep*—Phenomena necessary for restorative function; alterations include the spectrum of sleep disorders.

- *Sensation*—The ability to sense and distinguish internal and external stimuli; alterations include decreased sensation and pain.

- *Elimination*—Bodily excretion of waste products; alterations include bowel and bladder dysfunction secondary to nervous system disease.

- *Sexuality*—The ability to interact and maintain a sexual relationship; alterations include sexual dysfunction secondary to nervous system disease.

- *Self-care*—The ability to provide for one's basic needs; alterations include the inability to care for oneself.

- *Integrated regulation*—The interrelationship between the nervous system and other body systems; alterations include loss of regulatory control.

(Stewart-Amidei & Kunkel, 2000)

Historical Perspective on Neuroscience Nursing Standards and Evolution of Practice

In the mid-20th century and beyond, advances in medical treatment and healthcare technology led to the evolution of nursing specialties. Specialized education, training, and certification ensued in both traditional and newer areas of clinical practice, including neuroscience nursing. Neuroscience nursing was formalized as a specialty in 1968 with the formation of the American Association of Neurosurgical Nurses (AANN). In 1985, the organization's name was changed to the American Association of Neuroscience Nurses to better reflect the practice diversity of its members.

A statement of the standards of neurologic and neurosurgical nursing practice was first completed in 1977, and was approved by the executive committee of the ANA's division of medical-surgical nursing practice and AANN. A statement of neuroscience nursing's scope of practice was first completed in 1986 by the AANN Nursing Practice Committee. This document described the parameters of nursing practice for the specialty, identified the population served and practice settings, and distinguished qualifications of nurses in the specialty and the type of care rendered to patients. This description was useful to the neuroscience nurse in defining goals, and to the public for clarifying expectations.

In 1993, the standards and scope of practice statements were combined into a single document and updated, addressing the expanded options for neuroscience nursing in the 1990s. The third revision, *Scope and Standards of Neuroscience Nursing Practice,* issued in 2002, reflected practice evolution at the beginning of the new millennium. The borders of nursing practice have grown in recent years, with potential for continued change as healthcare reforms take shape. A renewed emphasis is placed on care of patients across the lifespan and a spectrum of health states rather than focusing on episodes of illness.

Neuroscience nursing practice has evolved along with clinical advances. Previously, neuroscience nursing care focused on symptom management and prevention of secondary complications. Although these approaches continue to be necessary, advances have offered new hope for persons with neurologic dysfunction. In recent decades, care of the patient with multiple sclerosis has evolved from symptomatic care to educating patients about administration of immunomodulating drugs. Neuroscience nurses can now help reduce deficits in stroke patients through the use of thrombolytic therapy and education geared toward early recognition of stroke symptoms. Advances in clinical monitoring, including intracranial pressure monitoring and brain tissue oxygenation monitoring, have allowed neuroscience nurses to become more skilled in applying data about neurologic function to the plan of care. Neuroscience nursing research findings have contributed to improved outcomes for children with seizures and for families of persons with brain tumors.

As neuroscience nursing evolved as a specialty, so did practice opportunities for APRNs. Increased availability of advanced education, combined with the shortage of primary care providers, need to improve quality of care, restricted residency hours, and promotion of cost-effective care, have led to increasing use of advanced practice nurses. The number of APRNs in neuroscience nursing has grown in recent decades, reflecting the complexity and diversity of the field. In 2009, work began on a scope of practice and standards document for advanced neuroscience nursing practice, which was published in 2010 (Stewart-Amidei et al., 2010). This fourth revision of *Neuroscience Nursing: Scope and Standards of Practice* is a collaboration of AANN and ANA, reflects an update to the 2002 neuroscience nursing scope and standards resource, and incorporates neuroscience advanced practice registered nursing scope and standards content.

Neuroscience Nursing's Scope and Standards of Practice

Description of the Scope of Neuroscience Nursing Practice

The specialty of neuroscience nursing has one scope of practice that encompasses a broad range of nursing practice and settings. This scope of practice statement describes who neuroscience nurses are and how they practice.

A neuroscience nurse is a registered nurse who provides care to individuals at risk for or with actual problems due to neurologic dysfunction, their families, and the communities in which they live. Neuroscience nurses provide care across the lifespan, from birth through death. Major categories of conditions that produce alterations of concern to neuroscience nurses include degenerative diseases (such as multiple sclerosis and Alzheimer's disease), tumors of the nervous system, neuromuscular diseases (such as myasthenia gravis), traumatic injury to the brain and spine, stroke and other cerebrovascular diseases, seizures, pain, diseases of the spine, movement disorders (such as Parkinson's disease and dystonia), and developmental problems of the nervous system. Neuroscience nurses also focus on prevention of nervous system dysfunction through health promotion, community education, and research.

No other specialty specifically addresses persons with neurologic dysfunction. The depth and breadth in which individual neuroscience nurses engage in the total scope of neuroscience nursing practice depends on their education, experience, role, and work environment, and is addressed in greater detail later in this document.

Neuroscience nursing is a learned specialty built on a core body of knowledge that reflects its dual components of science and art (Bader & Littlejohns, 2010). Neuroscience nursing requires judgment and skill based on principles of the biological, physical, psychological, behavioral, and social sciences with specific focus on neurologic function. Neuroscience nurses employ critical thinking to integrate objective data with knowledge gained from an assessment of the subjective experiences of patients. Neuroscience nurses use critical thinking to apply the best available evidence and research data to diagnosis and treatment. Neuroscience nurses continually evaluate quality and effectiveness of nursing practice and seek to optimize outcomes.

The Science of Neuroscience Nursing

The science of neuroscience nursing is based on an analytical framework of critical thinking comprised of assessment, diagnosis, identification of outcomes, planning, implementation, and evaluation, collectively known as the *nursing process*. These steps serve as the foundation of clinical decision-making and support evidence-based practice. Wherever they practice, neuroscience nurses use the nursing process and other types of critical thinking to respond to the needs of the populations they serve, and use strategies that support optimal outcomes most appropriate to the patient or situation, being mindful of resource utilization.

Neuroscience nurses as scientists rely on evidence to guide their policies and practices, but also as a way of quantifying the nurses' impact on the health outcomes of patients. An example of AANN leadership in this area is the development of the AANN Clinical Practice Guidelines series, which provides evidence-based directives for nurses caring for patients with problems such as traumatic brain injury or brain tumor.

Neuroscience nurses also generate new knowledge in their field through systematic research. In 1993, AANN established the Neuroscience Nursing Foundation, with the primary purpose of advancing the science and practice of neuroscience nursing. In 2011, updated strategies were proposed to meet this purpose (Di Iorio et al., 2011):

- Promote evidence-based practice to inform clinical decision-making

- Select strong research designs based on current research practices

- Develop and test nursing interventions

- Test theoretical or conceptual models for neuroscience nursing practice

- Build programs of research involving interdisciplinary teams

Research priorities identified include acute care outcomes, health promotion, end-of-life nursing care, quality-of-life improvements, and special population needs. Research in these areas is necessary to inform, distinguish, and advance neuroscience nursing practice.

The Art of Neuroscience Nursing

The art of neuroscience nursing is based on caring and respect for human dignity. A compassionate approach to patient care carries a mandate to provide that care competently. Competent care is provided and accomplished through both independent practice and partnerships. Collaboration may be with other colleagues or with the individuals seeking support or assistance with their healthcare needs. Central to neuroscience nursing practice is the art of caring, which is represented in the personal relationship that the nurse enters with the patient. The art of caring goes beyond the emotional connections of humans to the ability to respond to the human aspects of health and illness within the critical moment to promote healing within the context of social justice (Watson, 2008).

The art of neuroscience nursing embraces dynamic processes that affect the human person, including, for example, spirituality, healing, empathy, mutual respect, and compassion. These intangible aspects foster health. Neuroscience nursing embraces healing. Healing is fostered by compassion, helping, listening, mentoring, coaching, teaching, exploring, being present, supporting, touching, intuition, empathy, service, cultural competence, tolerance, acceptance, nurturing, mutually creating, and conflict resolution.

Neuroscience nursing focuses on the promotion and maintenance of health and the prevention or resolution of disease, illness, or disability. The nursing needs of human beings are identified from a holistic perspective and are met in the context of a culturally sensitive, caring, personal relationship. Neuroscience nursing includes the diagnosis and treatment of human responses to actual or potential health problems. Neuroscience nurses employ practices that are restorative, supportive, and promotive in nature.

- *Restorative* practices modify the impact of neurologic illness or disease.

- *Supportive* practices are oriented toward modification of relationships or the environment to support health.

- *Promotive* practices mobilize healthy patterns of living, foster personal and family development, and support self-defined goals of individuals, families, communities, and populations.

Development and Function of Nursing Standards

The standards of neuroscience nursing practice are authoritative statements of the duties that neuroscience nurses—regardless of role, population, or subspecialty served—are expected to competently perform (adapted from ANA, 2010a, p. 2). The standards published herein may be utilized as evidence of a legal standard of care and govern neuroscience nurses practicing within the role, population, and specialty governed by this document. The standards are subject to change with the dynamics of the neuroscience nursing specialty; as new patterns of professional practice are developed and accepted by neuroscience nurses, the education community, and the public; and as changes in societal trends occur. "Standards are subject to formal, periodic review and revision" (ANA, 2010a, p. 31).

This document includes 16 standards statements that provide the neuroscience nurse with a framework for outlining an expansive scope of practice. The language is intentionally broad and serves to paint an overall picture of practice. The standards statements become more effective, however, when viewed as a comprehensive and refined listing of expectations essential to practice without further development and explication. The roles and activities in which the neuroscience nurse is involved may be specific to the setting, and directed by state, institutional, or group practice requirements. Standard statements optimally inform nursing practice or the recipients of nursing care when tailored to the specifics of the focus or setting (ANA, 2010a).

Each standard statement is accompanied by several basic competencies. The competency statements in turn may be further specified according to the practice setting. Competencies are specific, measurable elements that interpret, explain, and facilitate practical use of a standard (ANA, 2010a). The competencies may be evidence of compliance with the individual standard but are not exhaustive, and depend on the circumstances. For example, the nurse may not be able to develop the plan of care (Standard 4, Planning) with or communicate it to the unresponsive patient who has no identified family caregiver.

Competencies may be used by neuroscience nursing professionals to appraise professional performance and identify content for academic and continuing education curricula. Neuroscience nurses can also use the competencies to inform others as to practice expectations.

The Nursing Process

Neuroscience nurses use the nursing process to deliver care. The nursing process is often conceptualized as having linear direction from assessment to diagnosis, outcomes identification, planning, implementation, and evaluation. However, these steps are often necessarily interrelated, as one step may inform another (Figure 1; ANA, 2010a).

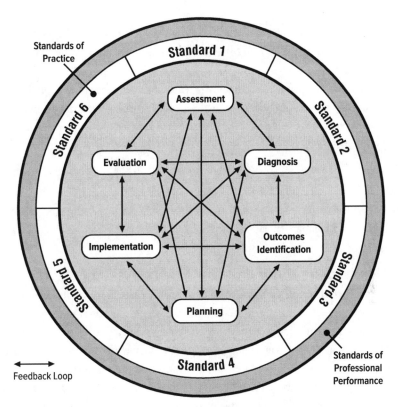

FIGURE 1. The Relationship of the Nursing Process
to Practice Standards (ANA, 2010a).

The Neuroscience Nursing Standards of Practice coincide with the steps of
the nursing process. The nursing process begins with assessment, with specific
attention focused on neurologic assessment. Data gathered from the neurologic
assessment are used to plan and implement nursing interventions specific to
the patient's neurologic dysfunction. Interventions may support bodily functions and promote healing and recovery of the acutely ill; enhance adaptation
to persistent neurologic deficits for the chronically ill; facilitate patient, family,
and significant other coping; and teach patients, families, and significant others
about disease processes, adaptation techniques, and therapies. The neuroscience nurse evaluates the outcomes of nursing care on an ongoing basis, and
revises the plan as necessary. Further, application of clinically relevant research

promotes evidence-based care and development of creative therapeutic nursing interventions to improve outcomes for patients with neurologic dysfunction.

Ethical principles are applied in any care rendered. Similarly, the Neuroscience Nursing Standards of Professional Performance relate to how the professional nurse adheres to the Neuroscience Nursing Standards of Practice, completes the nursing process, and addresses other practice issues and concerns (ANA, 2010a).

Tenets of Neuroscience Nursing Practice

Five tenets characterize contemporary neuroscience nursing practice, and are reflective of nursing practice as a whole:

1. Neuroscience nursing practice is individualized.

Neuroscience nursing practice respects diversity and is individualized to meet the unique needs of the patient. The *patient* is defined as the individual with or at risk for neurologic dysfunction, that individual's family, or a group, community, or population who is the focus of attention and to whom the neuroscience nurse is providing services as sanctioned by the state regulatory bodies. For example, the neuroscience nurse recognizes that each person with a brain tumor or stroke will present different signs, and care must be individualized according to identified needs.

2. Neuroscience nurses coordinate care by establishing partnerships.

Neuroscience registered nurses and APRNs establish partnerships with persons, families, communities, support systems, and other providers, utilizing in-person and electronic communication methods, to reach a shared goal of delivering health care. Collaborative, interprofessional team planning is based on recognition of each discipline's value and contributions, mutual trust, respect, open discussion, and shared decision-making. Neuroscience nurses frequently partner with other disciplines, such as physical therapy, occupational therapy, and speech therapy, to provide optimum care. Care may also be coordinated with other specialties, including pediatrics, psychiatry, or geriatrics. Knowledge gains in the genetics and immunology fields also require that neuroscience nurses work with these specialists.

3. Caring is central to the practice of neuroscience nursing.

Professional nursing promotes healing and health in a way that builds a relationship between the neuroscience nurse and patients (adapted from Watson, 2008). "Caring is a conscious judgment that manifests itself in concrete acts, interpersonally, verbally, and non-verbally" (Gallagher-Lepak & Kubsch, 2009, p. 171). Although caring for individuals, families, and populations is the key focus of neuroscience nursing, neuroscience registered nurses and APRNs additionally promote self-care, as well as care of the environment and society (Hagerty, Lynch-Sauer, Patusky, & Bouwsema, 1993). Neuroscience nurses communicate caring through touch, verbal communication, and their non-verbal behaviors.

4. Neuroscience registered nurses and APRNs use the nursing process to plan and provide individualized care to their patients.

Neuroscience registered nurses and APRNs use theoretical and evidence-based knowledge of human experiences and responses to advocate for and collaborate with patients in assessing, diagnosing, identifying outcomes, planning, implementing, and evaluating care. Nursing interventions are intended to produce beneficial effects, contribute to quality outcomes, and above all do no harm. "Nurses evaluate the effectiveness of their care in relation to identified outcomes and use evidence-based practice to improve care" (ANA, 2010a, pp. 4–5). Critical thinking underlies each step of the nursing, problem-solving, and decision-making processes. The nursing process is cyclical and dynamic, with each step informing both the previous step and the succeeding step. The nursing process is also patient centered, interpersonal and collaborative, and universally applicable.

5. A strong link exists between the professional work environment and neuroscience registered nurses' and APRNs' ability to provide quality patient care and achieve optimal patient outcomes.

Professional neuroscience registered nurses and APRNs have an ethical obligation to maintain and improve healthcare environments conducive to the provision of quality healthcare (ANA, 2001). Elements of a healthy work environment have been extensively studied and document the relationship between effective practice and quality of the work environment. Neuroscience registered nurses and APRNs must maintain and improve the healthcare environment for both nurses and patients in order to prevent injury and illness as well as promote health.

Healthy Work Environments for Neuroscience Nursing

Evidence demonstrates that negative, demoralizing, and unsafe conditions in the workplace, emanating from a physically or psychologically unhealthy environment, contribute to nursing errors, ineffective delivery of care, and conflict and stress among healthcare or other professionals and those they serve. The neuroscience nurse is expected to contribute toward the reduction or elimination of physical and psychological health risks in whatever setting employed, creating a healthy work environment.

The Institute of Medicine (IOM, 2004) reported that safety and quality problems exist when dedicated health professionals work within systems that neither prepare nor support them in achieving optimal patient care outcomes. Rapid changes, such as reimbursement modification and cost-containment efforts, new healthcare technologies, and changes in the healthcare workforce, have influenced the work and work environment of all nurses. Concentration on key aspects of the work environment, encompassing people, physical places, and tools, can enhance healthcare working conditions and improve safety. Key aspects include utilizing transformational leadership and evidence-based care management; maximizing workforce capability; creating and sustaining a culture of safety and research; evaluating work space design and redesign to prevent and mitigate errors; addressing potential pollutants in the work environment; and promoting the effective use of telecommunications.

Creating and maintaining a healthy work environment requires effort. The establishment and maintenance of a healthy work environment requires *all* nurses, not only neuroscience nurses, to:

- Be proficient in skilled communication

- Foster true collaboration with partners across all disciplines

- Be effective decision-makers regarding policy, in directing and evaluating clinical care, and in leading organizations

- Ensure appropriate staffing that matches nurse competencies to patient needs

- Foster meaningful recognition of the value of self and others

- Embrace the role of a leader in creating and sustaining a healthy work environment

(AACN, 2005)

The Magnet Recognition Program® (ANCC, 2008) also addresses the professional work environment, requiring that Magnet®-designated facilities adhere to the model components of transformational leadership, structured empowerment, exemplary professional practice, new knowledge, innovation and improvements, and empirical quality results.

These collective principles of a healthy employment environment apply to neuroscience nurses who work in any healthcare environment. This requires the neuroscience nurse to collaborate often and well; to communicate the important contributions of nursing to the health and well-being of those with neurologic dysfunction; and to assume leadership roles in settings where they are employed.

Issues specific to a healthy work environment for neuroscience nurses relate to the nature of the phenomena encountered in practice. While ethical concerns exist in all areas of nursing practice, neuroscience nurses may more frequently encounter issues that create moral distress. Persons who are diagnosed as brain dead or with futile outcomes present the most challenging of ethical concerns to both the nurses who care for them and their families. Care may be withheld or withdrawn, changing the focus from cure to comfort. Neuroscience nurses may participate in unit discussions, ethics consults, and ethics committees to help manage moral distress.

Persons with neurologic dysfunction are often unable to move independently and may require a great deal of physical assistance, thereby placing the neuroscience nurse at risk for injury. Neuroscience nurses can use special equipment, including mechanical lifts and back braces, or services such as lift teams to protect themselves. Persons with neurologic dysfunction may present unfavorable behaviors that can injure themselves, family members, or health care staff. Within their work environment, neuroscience nurses promote safety by observing for escalating violent behaviors, working as a team to defuse these violent patient behaviors, and educating family members and coworkers about how to best deal with these safety concerns.

Model of Professional Practice Regulation

In 2006, the Model of Professional Nursing Practice Regulation (Figure 2) emerged from ANA work and informed the discussions of specialty nursing and advanced practice neuroscience nurse practice. *Neuroscience Nursing: Scope and Standards of Practice* is derived from this model.

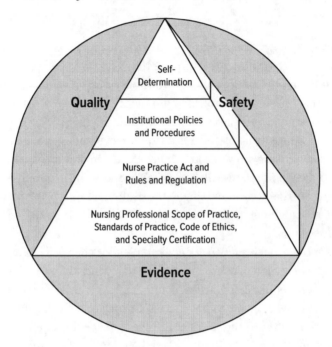

FIGURE 2. Model of Professional Nursing Practice Regulation (Styles, Schumann, Bickford, & White, 2008).

The lowest level in the model represents the responsibility of professional and specialty nursing organizations to their members and the public to define the scope and standards of practice for neuroscience nursing. The next level up the pyramid represents the regulation provided by the nurse practice acts, rules, and regulations in the pertinent licensing jurisdictions. Institutional policies and procedures provide further considerations in the regulation of nursing practice for the neuroscience nurse and advanced practice neuroscience nurse. Note that the highest level is that of self-determination by the neuroscience nurse after consideration of all the other levels of input about professional nursing practice regulation. The outcome is safe, quality, and evidence-based practice.

Overview of the Standards of Neuroscience Nursing Practice

The Standards of Neuroscience Nursing Practice are comprised of the Standards of Practice and the Standards of Professional Performance.

STANDARDS OF PRACTICE FOR NEUROSCIENCE NURSING

The Standards of Practice describe a competent level of nursing care as demonstrated by the critical thinking model known as the nursing process. The nursing process includes the components of assessment, diagnosis, outcomes identification, planning, implementation, and evaluation, with a focus on the patient with actual or potential neurologic dysfunction. Accordingly, the nursing process encompasses significant actions taken by neuroscience nurses and forms the foundation of the nurse's decision-making.

STANDARD 1. ASSESSMENT

The neuroscience registered nurse collects comprehensive data pertinent to the patient's health and/or the situation.

STANDARD 2. DIAGNOSIS

The neuroscience registered nurse analyzes assessment data in determining diagnoses or issues.

STANDARD 3. OUTCOMES IDENTIFICATION

The neuroscience registered nurse identifies expected outcomes for a plan individualized to the patient.

STANDARD 4. PLANNING

The neuroscience registered nurse develops a plan of care that prescribes strategies and alternatives to attain expected outcomes.

STANDARD 5. IMPLEMENTATION

The neuroscience registered nurse implements the identified plan.

STANDARD 5A. COORDINATION OF CARE

The neuroscience registered nurse coordinates care delivery.

STANDARD 5B. HEALTH TEACHING AND HEALTH PROMOTION

The neuroscience registered nurse employs strategies to promote health and a safe environment for the patient with actual or potential neurologic dysfunction.

STANDARD 5C. CONSULTATION

The neuroscience advanced practice registered nurse provides consultation to influence the identified plan for the patient, enhance the abilities of others, and effect change.

STANDARD 5D. PRESCRIPTIVE AUTHORITY AND TREATMENT

The neuroscience advanced practice registered nurse uses prescriptive authority, procedures, referrals, treatments, and therapies in accordance with state and federal laws and regulations.

STANDARD 6. EVALUATION

The neuroscience registered nurse evaluates the progress toward attainment of expected outcomes.

STANDARDS OF PROFESSIONAL PERFORMANCE
FOR NEUROSCIENCE NURSING

The Standards of Professional Performance describe a competent level of behavior in the professional role, including activities related to ethics, education, evidence-based practice and research, quality of practice, communication, leadership, collaboration, professional practice evaluation, resource utilization, and environmental health. All neuroscience registered nurses and APRNs are expected to engage in professional role activities, including leadership, appropriate to their education and position. Neuroscience registered nurses and APRNs are accountable for their professional actions to themselves, their patients, their peers, and ultimately to society.

STANDARD 7. ETHICS

The neuroscience registered nurse practices ethically.

STANDARD 8. EDUCATION

The neuroscience registered nurse attains knowledge and competence that reflect current nursing practice.

STANDARD 9. EVIDENCE-BASED PRACTICE AND RESEARCH
The neuroscience registered nurse integrates evidence and research findings into practice.

STANDARD 10. QUALITY OF PRACTICE
The neuroscience registered nurse contributes to quality nursing practice.

STANDARD 11. COMMUNICATION
The neuroscience registered nurse communicates effectively in a variety of formats in all areas of practice.

STANDARD 12. LEADERSHIP
The neuroscience registered nurse demonstrates leadership in the professional practice setting and the profession.

STANDARD 13. COLLABORATION
The neuroscience registered nurse collaborates with the patient, family, and others in the conduct of nursing practice.

STANDARD 14. PROFESSIONAL PRACTICE EVALUATION
The neuroscience registered nurse evaluates her or his own nursing practice in relation to professional practice standards and guidelines, relevant statutes, rules, and regulations.

STANDARD 15. RESOURCE UTILIZATION
The neuroscience registered nurse utilizes appropriate resources to plan and provide nursing services that are safe, effective, and financially responsible.

STANDARD 16. ENVIRONMENTAL HEALTH
The neuroscience registered nurse practices in an environmentally safe and healthy manner.

Professional Competence in Neuroscience Nursing Practice

The public has a right to expect neuroscience registered nurses and APRNs to demonstrate professional competence throughout their careers. Neuroscience registered nurses and APRNs are individually responsible and accountable for maintaining professional competence. It is the nursing profession's responsibility to shape and guide any process for assuring neuroscience nurse competence. Regulatory agencies define minimal standards of competence to protect the public. The employer is responsible and accountable to provide a practice environment conducive to competent practice. Assurance of competence is the shared responsibility of the profession, individual nurses, professional organizations, credentialing and certification entities, regulatory agencies, employers, and other key stakeholders (ANA, 2008).

AANN believes that in the practice of neuroscience nursing, competence can be defined, measured, and evaluated. No single evaluation method or tool can guarantee competence. Competence is situational and dynamic; it is both an outcome and an ongoing process. Context determines what competencies are necessary.

DEFINITIONS AND CONCEPTS RELATED TO NEUROSCIENCE NURSING COMPETENCE

A number of terms are central to the discussion of competence:

- An individual who demonstrates "competence" is performing at an expected level.

- A *competency* is an expected level of performance that integrates knowledge, skills, abilities, and judgment.

- The integration of knowledge, skills, abilities, and judgment occurs in formal, informal, and reflective learning experiences.

- Knowledge encompasses thinking; understanding of science and humanities; professional standards of practice; and insights gained from context, practical experiences, personal capabilities, and leadership performance.

- Skills include psychomotor, communication, interpersonal, and diagnostic skills.

- *Ability* is the capacity to act effectively. It requires listening, integrity, knowledge of one's strengths and weaknesses, positive self-regard, emotional intelligence, and openness to feedback.

- Judgment includes critical thinking, problem-solving, ethical reasoning, and decision-making.

■ *Formal learning* most often occurs in structured, academic, and professional development practice environments, whereas *informal learning* can be described as experiential insights gained in work, community, home, and other settings.

■ *Reflective learning* represents the recurrent, thoughtful personal self-assessment, analysis, and synthesis of strengths and opportunities for improvement. Such insights should lead to the creation of a specific plan for professional development and may become part of one's professional portfolio (ANA, 2008).

COMPETENCE AND COMPETENCY IN NEUROSCIENCE NURSING PRACTICE

Competent neuroscience nursing practice can be influenced by the nature of the situation, which includes consideration of the setting, resources, and the person. Situations can either enhance or detract from the neuroscience nurse's ability to perform. Neuroscience registered nurses and APRNs influence factors that facilitate and enhance competent practice. Similarly, neuroscience registered nurses and APRNs seek to deal with barriers that constrain competent practice. The expected level of performance will vary depending upon context and the selected competence framework or model.

The ability to perform at the expected level requires a process of lifelong learning. Neuroscience registered nurses and APRNs must continually reassess their competencies and identify needs for additional knowledge, skills, personal growth, and integrative learning experiences.

EVALUATING COMPETENCE

Competence in neuroscience nursing practice must be evaluated by the individual nurse (self-assessment), nurse peers, and nurses in the roles of supervisor, coach, mentor, or preceptor. In addition, other aspects of neuroscience nursing performance may be evaluated by professional colleagues and patients.

Competence can be evaluated by using tools that capture objective and subjective data about the individual's knowledge base and actual performance and are appropriate for the specific situation and the desired outcome of the competence evaluation. "However, no single evaluation tool or method can guarantee competence" (ANA, 2008, p. 6).

Professional Neuroscience Nurses Today

STATISTICAL SNAPSHOT

Neuroscience registered nurses and APRNs may choose membership in the organization supporting the specialty, the American Association of Neuroscience Nurses (AANN). Not all neuroscience registered nurses and APRNs are members of this organization. Therefore, statistics on neuroscience registered nurses and APRNs are limited to AANN membership, comprising about 4,700 registered nurses and APRNs. AANN members primarily work in academic medical centers, but often work in community hospitals as well as in ambulatory or rehabilitation settings, or in private practices. Primary practice areas are medical-surgical and critical care, although some work in outpatient and perioperative areas. Neuroscience registered nurses and APRNs work with patients across the lifespan, as neurologic dysfunction may occur at any age. Neuroscience registered nurses and APRNs in specialty practice represent the full spectrum from novice to expert.

The continuation of the profession depends on the education of nurses, appropriate organization of nursing services, continued expansion of nursing knowledge, and the development and adoption of policies. Such initiatives demand that neuroscience nurses be adequately prepared for specialty practice. Neuroscience registered nurses and APRNs collaborate, consult, and serve as liaisons, bridging the role of the professional neuroscience registered nurse with that of other professionals, and subsequently help to delineate nursing's role in society.

LICENSURE AND EDUCATION OF NEUROSCIENCE REGISTERED NURSES

The neuroscience nurse is licensed as a registered nurse and authorized by a state, commonwealth, or territory to practice nursing. Licensure of the health-care professions is established by each jurisdiction to protect the public safety and authorize the practice of the profession. Because of this, the requirements for registered nurse licensure and advanced practice nursing vary widely.

The neuroscience registered nurse is educationally prepared for competent practice at the beginning level upon graduation from an accredited school of nursing and is qualified by national examination for registered nurse licensure. Through orientation, continuing education, guided practice, and mentorship, nurses develop the specialized body of knowledge and experience that characterizes neuroscience nursing practice. Credentialing is one form of acknowledging such specialized knowledge and experience.

Credentialing organizations may mandate specific nursing educational requirements, as well as timely demonstrations of knowledge and experience in specialty practice. Registered nurses who have worked in neuroscience nursing for at least two years may choose to test their proficiency in neuroscience nursing to become a certified neuroscience registered nurse (CNRN). Ongoing certification may be retained either through continuing education or retesting, and appropriate documentation must be maintained. The neuroscience registered nurse may also seek and maintain other professional certifications.

The neuroscience registered nurse is educated in the art and science of nursing, with the goal of helping individuals and groups attain, maintain, and restore health whenever possible. Experienced nurses may become proficient in one or more practice areas or roles. These nurses may concentrate on patient care in clinical nursing practice specialties. Others influence nursing and support the direct care rendered to patients by those professional nurses in clinical practice.

Neuroscience registered nurses who have not acquired a baccalaureate degree in nursing are encouraged to earn this degree. Neuroscience registered nurses may pursue advanced academic studies to prepare for specialization in practice. Educational requirements vary by specialty and educational program. New models for educational preparation are evolving in response to the changing healthcare, education, and regulatory practice environments. All neuroscience registered nurses have the professional responsibility to maintain their competence in practice through ongoing skill development and continuing education. AANN offers continuing education through professional conferences and through its journal, *Journal of Neuroscience Nursing*. In some states, continuing education is tied to relicensure.

NEUROSCIENCE ADVANCED PRACTICE REGISTERED NURSES

The need to ensure patient safety and access to advance practice registered nurses, by aligning education, accreditation, licensure, and certification, is delineated in *Consensus Model for APRN Regulation: Licensure, Accreditation, Certification, and Education* (APRN Joint Dialogue Group [JDG], 2008). The APRN Joint Dialogue Group (2008) defines the advanced practice registered nurse as having:

- Completed an accredited graduate-level education program with preparation in one of the four recognized APRN roles;

■ Passed a national certification examination that measures APRN competencies;

■ Acquired advanced clinical knowledge and skills preparing him or her to provide direct care to patients, as well as a component of indirect care;

■ A practice that builds on the competencies of the registered nurse;

■ Educational preparation to assume responsibility and accountability for health promotion and/or maintenance as well as the assessment, diagnosis, and management of patient problems, which includes the use and prescription of pharmacologic and nonpharmacologic interventions;

■ Clinical experience of sufficient depth and breadth to reflect the intended license; and

■ Obtained a license to practice as an APRN in one of the four APRN roles: certified registered nurse anesthetist (CRNA), certified nurse midwife (CNM), clinical nurse specialist (CNS), or certified nurse practitioner (CNP).

The AANN supports the four requirements necessary for regulation of the advanced practice role: licensure, accreditation, certification, and education (APRN JDG, 2008). *Advanced Practice Registered Nurse* is a regulatory title and in neuroscience nursing includes the roles of either clinical nurse specialist (CNS) or nurse practitioner (NP). State laws and regulations further define criteria for licensure for the designated scopes of practice.

The neuroscience advanced practice registered nurse has a specialized body of knowledge and expanded clinical skills acquired at the graduate level, with the master's degree as the minimum requirement for entry into advanced practice (APRN JDG, 2008). Advanced practice certification via examination through the appropriate nationally recognized organization is a requirement for licensure in most states. The American Nurses Credentialing Center offers multiple certification examinations for nurse practitioners and clinical nurse specialists, in addition to other advanced practice examinations (ANCC, 2008). Specialty nursing certification exams for advanced practice, such as those offered through the Oncology Nursing Certification Corporation, the Pediatric Nursing Credentialing Board, and the American Association of Critical Care Nurses Certification Corporation, may also be acceptable for licensure.

Roles and Responsibilities of Neuroscience Registered Nurses

Neuroscience registered nurse responsibilities focus on the unique problems of patients with neurologic dysfunction, and the primary role is direct care delivery. Beyond direct delivery of care, the neuroscience nurse may assume a variety of roles, such as educator, administrator, researcher, consultant, advocate, and clinical expert. Each role is based upon specific clinical expertise and education. Basic nursing role titles may include staff nurse with varying degrees of advancement.

Neuroscience registered nurse responsibilities focus on the patient with neurologic dysfunction and include:

- Providing age-appropriate and culturally and linguistically appropriate care

- Maintaining a safe environment

- Educating patients about healthy practices and treatment modalities

- Assuring continuity of care

- Coordinating the care across settings and among caregivers

- Managing information

- Communicating effectively

Specific responsibilities may be specified by the setting where the neuroscience nurse is employed.

Professionalism is demonstrated by assuming accountability for maintaining excellence in practice through self-motivated ventures, as well as collaborative efforts with other nursing colleagues, organizations, and intraprofessional associates. Participation in the specialty's certification process further identifies the nurse's commitment to excellence in neuroscience nursing practice.

Roles and Responsibilities of Neuroscience Advanced Practice Registered Nurses

Expert clinical practice is the hallmark of advanced practice nursing. Clinical practice involves assessment, diagnosis, and management of patient problems, as well as health promotion. Primary generic responsibilities, regardless of specialty, identify the following responsibilities of the APRN (APRN JDG, 2008):

- Plans and coordinates interventions from a multidisciplinary perspective

- Functions across the healthcare system and works with diverse populations

- Initiates and facilitates quality improvement initiatives

- Facilitates, conducts, and promotes utilization of research activities in practice

- Develops education strategies and evaluates effectiveness of educational interventions

- Recommends and influences social and healthcare policies

- Provides consultation to improve care

- Applies legal and ethical standards to complex situations

Each of these responsibilities may be directly applied into specialty practice by the neuroscience APRN (Villanueva et al., 2008). Interventions may occur from an independent or collaborative decision-making position. Specific neuroscience APRN activities may be influenced by workforce fluctuations, development of related healthcare specialties, geographic and economic disparities, economic incentives, and consumer demand. There are many diverse statutes (state, federal, community) and institutional guidelines that govern APRNs. For those APRNs who are required to practice within a contractual agreement, protocols may be collaboratively developed that address specific responsibilities and expectations (Yeager, Shaw, Casavant, & Burns, 2006).

Neuroscience Nurse Practice Settings

Neuroscience registered nurses practice in a wide range of settings, caring for patients with biopsychosocial alterations as a result of nervous system dysfunction and for their families or significant others. There are multiple practice sites for neuroscience patients, including hospitals, outpatient settings, private practice, academic institutions, research facilities, rehabilitation centers, and community settings. Patient care may have a specific disease focus, such as neuro-oncology; a specialty focus, such as neurosurgery; or a problem focus, such as chronic pain management. Patient care may be provided across the lifespan, or within a specific age group (children or older adults).

Neuroscience APRNs work in a variety of settings, demonstrate specific competencies unique to neuroscience nursing, and have a broad scope of responsibilities. The neuroscience APRN may practice collaboratively in any of the settings previously described. The following are examples of advanced practice applications, but are by no means limited to these settings. The neuroscience APRN may practice in the neurosurgery intensive care unit, providing direct patient care while mentoring staff nurses and orienting new graduates. Another neuroscience APRN may have pediatric neurosurgery as the specialty, performing preoperative and postoperative assessments of children and/or providing direct and indirect care to children in the ICU with complex neurosurgical needs (e.g., traumatic brain injury, craniotomy for tumor resection, cranial vault remodeling, and neonates with myelomeningocele). Another neuroscience APRN may practice in the clinic setting, providing specialized care to older adult patients with movement disorders such as Parkinson's disease or myasthenia gravis, or manage care for both inpatients and outpatients, or provide stroke screening and implement stroke prevention initiatives. Another neuroscience APRN may work with a neuro-oncology team, coordinating radiation, chemotherapy, and surgical interventions—all the while helping the patient navigate hospital systems. The neuroscience APRN working in the perioperative area conducts assessments, writes orders, and assists the neurosurgical team.

In all of the identified settings, levels of practice, and roles, the primary intent is to care for, support, teach, and serve as an advocate for the patient with neurologic dysfunction. The goal of all intervention in neuroscience nursing practice is consistent with and flows from that of the entire nursing profession: to provide the highest quality of care to patients and achieve a state of wellness consistent with the quality of life desired by the patient, which may include a peaceful and dignified death.

Neuroscience Nursing's Societal and Ethical Dimensions

Neuroscience nursing is responsive to the changing needs of society and the expanding knowledge base of its theoretical and scientific domains. One of neuroscience nursing's objectives is to achieve positive patient outcomes that maximize quality of life across the entire lifespan. Neuroscience registered nurses and APRNs facilitate the interprofessional and comprehensive care provided by healthcare professionals, paraprofessionals, and volunteers. In other instances, neuroscience registered nurses and APRNs engage in consultation with other colleagues to inform decision-making and planning to meet patient needs. Neuroscience registered nurses and APRNs often participate in interprofessional teams in which the overlapping skills complement each member's individual efforts. All nursing practice, regardless of specialty, role, or setting, is fundamentally independent practice. Neuroscience registered nurses and APRNs are accountable for nursing judgments made and actions taken in the course of their nursing practice. Therefore, neuroscience registered nurses and APRNs are responsible for assessing individual competence and are committed to the process of lifelong learning. Neuroscience registered nurses and APRNs develop and maintain current knowledge and skills through formal and continuing education and seek certification when it is available in their areas of practice.

Neuroscience registered nurses and APRNs are bound by the same professional code of ethics (ANA, 2001) that guides all nurses. Neuroscience registered nurses and APRNs regulate themselves as individuals through a collegial process of peer review of practice. Peer evaluation fosters the refinement of knowledge, skills, and clinical decision-making at all levels and in all areas of clinical practice. Self-regulation by the profession of nursing assures quality of performance, which is the heart of nursing's social contract (ANA, 2010b).

Neuroscience registered nurses, neuroscience APRNs, and their professional colleagues exchange knowledge and ideas about how to deliver high-quality health care, resulting in constantly changing professional practice boundaries. True collaboration involves recognition of the expertise of others within and outside one's profession and consultation with and referral to specialized providers when appropriate. Collaboration also involves some shared functions and a common focus on one overall mission. By necessity, neuroscience nursing's scope of practice has flexible boundaries.

Neuroscience registered nurses and APRNs regularly evaluate safety, effectiveness, and cost in the planning and delivery of nursing care. Nurses recognize that resources are limited and unequally distributed, and that the potential for better access to care requires innovative approaches, such as treating patients remotely. As members of a profession, neuroscience registered nurses and APRNs work toward equitable distribution and availability of healthcare services throughout the nation and the world.

Ethical dimensions of neuroscience nursing practice are influenced by the nature of the phenomena that form the framework of neuroscience nursing. Patients cared for by neuroscience nurses may have altered responsiveness or language impairments that render them vulnerable and unable to speak up or otherwise communicate about their needs. Neuroscience nurses may serve as patient advocates and play an important role in facilitating surrogate decision-making on the patient's behalf. Encouraging patients to formulate advance directives allows patients to communicate their wishes when they become otherwise unable to do so.

The potential for irreversible brain injury or progressive neurologic deterioration in the population served by neuroscience nurses poses additional ethical concerns. Neuroscience nurses anticipate these problems and actively participate in discussions about withholding or withdrawal of care, preparing patients and families to address these issues as well. For example, when working with a patient with amyotrophic lateral sclerosis, the neuroscience nurse may participate in a discussion with the patient and family about the option of withholding intubation for respiratory distress, or explain the life support withdrawal process to the family of a patient pronounced brain dead. Patients with neurologic dysfunction may be left with persistent deficits. Neuroscience nurses also play an integral role in determining the need for rehabilitation and assuring access to restorative care.

Continued Commitment to the Profession

A continued commitment to the nursing profession requires neuroscience registered nurses and APRNs to remain involved in continuous learning and strengthening of individual practice within varied practice settings. This may include civic activities; membership in and support of professional associations, such as AANN; collective bargaining; and workplace advocacy. Neuroscience nurses promote the health of the individual and society regardless of cultural background, value system, religious belief, gender, sexual identity, or disability. Neuroscience nurses commit to their profession by utilizing their skills, knowledge, and abilities to act as visionaries, promoting safe practice environments, and supporting resourceful, accessible, and cost-effective delivery of health care to serve the ever-changing needs of the population. Neuroscience nurses are also committed to the advancement of their specialty through nursing research.

Professional Trends and Issues

Neuroscience nursing is evolving and will continue to do so, in conjunction with technological advances, greater scientific understanding, and a rapidly growing research base. Nursing has moved from an era of needing only to provide good, safe, physical care to the patient with severe neurologic dysfunction to the era of explicit incorporation of science and research into care. An example of this is the early treatment of stroke. Ten years ago, stroke care consisted of supportive and rehabilitative care only. It is now possible to reverse stroke deficits with early intervention, and neuroscience nurses at all levels of practice play a key role in this process.

Neuroscience registered nurses and APRNs are increasingly involved in research activities, not just as consumers, but also as independent or collaborative researchers. Advances in the various branches of science, such as neurogenetics, are rapidly changing the face of neuroscience nursing practice. Genetics may broaden treatment options, and nurses must be aware not only of the clinical implications of this, but of the ethical implications as well. Complementary and alternative medicine (CAM) options are expanding care further. Neuroscience registered nurses and APRNs are challenged to keep abreast of developments in CAM and integrative health strategies, and guide their patients in its use. Nursing interactions are moving beyond the traditional settings into novel areas such as industry, legal practice, insurance, and social service areas, and neuroscience nurses are encouraged to explore new venues that utilize their expertise.

The healthcare industry has been challenged to improve patient safety, patient and practitioner satisfaction, patient outcomes, and the profitability of the healthcare organization (Unruh, 2008). Patient safety will remain in the forefront of neuroscience nursing practice. The value of neuroscience nurses in patient safety and positive patient outcomes in hospital settings is well demonstrated (Kane, Shamilyan, Mueller, Duval, & Wilt, 2007). Employers are correcting workplace problems in an attempt to retain nurses. Safe patient handling, shift and scheduling options, integration of technology supports into practice, and alternative roles in the healthcare setting have enabled nurses to remain in the workplace.

A major impact on the scope of practice in neuroscience nursing is the changing healthcare delivery system. Societal, economic, and political pressures are driving the development of less costly means to meet the healthcare needs of the public. One way neuroscience nurses can be intimately involved in this process is by using advanced practice nurses to deliver care. Neuroscience APRNs, with their expanded knowledge base and expertise, can provide high-quality care in a more cost-effective manner (Holleman, Johnson, & Frim, 2010; Mills, Bachmann, Campbell, Hine, & McGowan, 1999). One example of this is a nurse-managed seizure clinic. Neuroscience APRNs can also function as consultants to registered nurses and other healthcare team members. Collaboration, along with effective use of resources, cost containment, increased participation by recipients of care, timely achievement of goals, and continuity of care, is critical to the future of neuroscience nursing as well as other healthcare systems.

The changing healthcare market will also have an impact on the practice of neuroscience nursing. As the population of the United States ages, chronic illness will predominate, and a shift in care delivery and focus from acute to chronic illness will be necessary. Neuroscience registered nurses and APRNs are challenged to redirect their practice and educators are challenged to meet the demand for practitioners. The focus of healthcare providers is evolving to address prevention and problem management across the lifespan, rather than focusing on episodic care alone.

The need for healthcare reform is a major concern. A reformed healthcare system focused on primary care, prevention, and chronic disease management can alleviate the financial and social costs of treating preventable and chronic diseases. Interprofessional teams and coordination of care across the illness trajectory will be key components in the new system, arenas in which neuroscience nurses are familiar and have demonstrated their value.

Neuroscience registered nurses and APRNs are positioned to play key roles in reforming and restructuring the care delivery system. A major shift from inpatient to outpatient care settings is occurring. More expanded roles in community-based programs are developing. Neuroscience registered nurses and APRNs are encouraged to support and participate in the "medical home" ("healthcare home") model for care management. Neuroscience APRNs should also be utilized to the fullest extent of their scope of practice consistent with education and competencies.

As healthcare reform evolves, nurses may experience greater opportunities to function within their full scope of practice across various settings. A reformed healthcare system will provide incentives and financial support for utilizing nurses in various roles and promoting a full scope of practice, and eliminate the current payment practices that may create barriers to innovative and effective models of practice and care delivery.

Nursing as a profession continues to face dilemmas regarding entry into practice, the autonomy of advanced practice, continued competence, multistate licensure, and the appropriate educational credentials for professional certification. Neuroscience registered nurses and APRNs have a professional responsibility to maintain competence in their area of practice. Employers who provide opportunities for professional development and continuing education promote a positive practice environment in which nurses can maintain and enhance skills and competencies. Critical to the future of neuroscience nursing is the ability to recruit an adequate number of nurses to the specialty, as well as to retain those who are currently practicing.

Technology offers a better work environment for neuroscience registered nurses and APRNs when designed and implemented in a manner that supports nurses' work. These work environments can include conventional locations— hospitals, clinics, and patient homes—as well as virtual spaces such as online discussion groups, e-mail, interactive video, and virtual interaction. Ideally, technology eliminates redundancy and duplication of documentation; reduces errors; eliminates interruptions for missing supplies, equipment, and medications; and eases access to data, thereby allowing the neuroscience registered nurse and APRN more time with the patient (IOM, 2009). The incorporation of technologies, however, is not without risk, and demands diligence by neuroscience nurses to consider the impact on the scope of neuroscience nursing practice and the ethical implications for patients as well as the nurse.

Regardless of the practice venue, over the next decade, neuroscience registered nurses and APRNs will continue to partner with others to advance the nation's health through collaborative initiatives. As practice changes evolve, neuroscience registered nurses and APRNs will be at the forefront. As neuroscience registered nurses and APRNs address these challenges, the major responsibility of neuroscience nursing will remain the realm of human responses to actual or potential health problems secondary to nervous system dysfunction.

Summary of the Scope of Neuroscience Nursing Practice

The dynamic nature of the healthcare practice environment and the growing body of nursing research provide both the impetus and the opportunity for nursing to ensure competent nursing practice in all settings for all patients and to promote ongoing professional development that enhances the quality of nursing practice (ANA, 2010a, p. 30). *Neuroscience Nursing: Scope and Standards of Practice* assists that process by delineating the professional scope and standards and responsibilities of all professional neuroscience nurses, regardless of setting. As such, it can serve as a basis for:

- Position recruitment announcement

- Position description creation

- New employee orientation

- Performance appraisal/evaluation

- Agency policy, protocol, and procedure development

- Competency identification and development

- Education of individuals regarding the role of neuroscience nurses

- Quality improvement systems and/or program evaluation efforts

- Development and evaluation of school nursing service delivery systems and organizational structures

- Educational offerings

- Database development, data collection, and research

- Establishment of a legal standard

- Healthcare reimbursement and financing methodologies

- Regulatory review and revision

Standards of Neuroscience Nursing Practice

The standards published herein may be used as evidence of the standard of care, with the understanding that application of the standards is context dependent. The standards are subject to change with the dynamics of the nursing profession, as new patterns of professional practice are developed and accepted by the nursing profession and the public. In addition, specific conditions and clinical circumstances may also affect the application of the standards at a given time (e.g., during a natural disaster). The standards are subject to formal periodic review and revision.

The competencies that accompany each standard may serve as evidence of compliance with the corresponding standard. The list of competencies is not exhaustive. Whether a particular standard or competency applies depends upon the context.

Standards of Practice for Neuroscience Nursing

Standard 1. Assessment

The neuroscience registered nurse collects comprehensive data pertinent to the patient's health and/or the situation.

COMPETENCIES

The neuroscience registered nurse:

- Collects comprehensive data, including but not limited to physical, functional, psychosocial, emotional, cognitive, sexual, cultural, age-related, environmental, spiritual/transpersonal, and economic assessments, in a systematic and ongoing process while honoring the uniqueness of the individual.

- Elicits the patient's values, preferences, expressed needs, and knowledge of the healthcare situation.

- Involves the patient, family, and other healthcare providers as appropriate, in holistic data collection.

- Identifies barriers (e.g., psychosocial, literacy, financial, cultural) to effective communication and makes appropriate adaptations.

- Recognizes the impact of personal attitudes, values, and beliefs.

- Assesses family dynamics and impact on patient health and wellness.

- Prioritizes data collection based on the patient's immediate condition, or the anticipated needs of the patient or situation.

- Uses appropriate evidence-based assessment techniques, instruments, and tools.

- Synthesizes available data, information, and knowledge relevant to the situation to identify patterns and variances.

- Applies ethical, legal, and privacy guidelines and policies to the collection, maintenance, use, and dissemination of data and information.

- Recognizes the patient as the authority on his or her own health by honoring the patient's care preferences.

- Documents relevant assessment data in a confidential, accessible, and retrievable format.

ADDITIONAL COMPETENCIES FOR THE
NEUROSCIENCE ADVANCED PRACTICE REGISTERED NURSE
The neuroscience advanced practice registered nurse:

- Utilizes advanced assessment techniques, incorporating technological data and diagnostic information where appropriate.

- Initiates and interprets diagnostic tests and procedures relevant to the patient's current status.

- Identifies system and personnel needs in the clinical environment that influence patient outcomes.

- Assesses the effect of interactions among individuals, family, community, and social systems on health and illness.

Standard 2. Diagnosis

The neuroscience registered nurse analyzes assessment data in determining diagnoses or issues.

COMPETENCIES

The neuroscience registered nurse:

- Derives diagnoses or issues from assessment data.

- Validates the diagnoses or issues with the patient, family, and other healthcare providers when possible and appropriate.

- Identifies actual or potential risks to the patient's health and safety or barriers to health, which may include, but are not limited to, interpersonal, systematic, or environmental circumstances.

- Uses standardized classification systems and clinical decision support tools, when available, in identifying diagnoses.

- Documents diagnoses or issues in a manner that facilitates determination of the expected outcomes and plan.

ADDITIONAL COMPETENCIES FOR THE NEUROSCIENCE ADVANCED PRACTICE REGISTERED NURSE

The neuroscience advanced practice registered nurse:

- Systematically compares and contrasts clinical findings with normal and abnormal variations and developmental events in formulating a differential diagnosis.

- Utilizes complex data and information obtained during interview, examination, and diagnostic processes in identifying diagnoses.

- Assists staff in developing and maintaining competence in the diagnostic process.

- Documents diagnoses in a manner that facilitates communication among the interprofessional team.

Standard 3. Outcomes Identification

The neuroscience registered nurse identifies expected outcomes for a plan individualized to the patient.

COMPETENCIES

The neuroscience registered nurse:

- Considers associated risks, benefits, costs, expected trajectory of the condition, and clinical expertise when formulating expected outcomes.

- Derives culturally appropriate expected outcomes from the diagnoses.

- Modifies outcomes in response to changing needs or condition of the patient.

- Ensures that outcomes are measurable, provide direction for continuity of care, and include an appropriate time frame for achievement.

- Formulates outcomes in collaboration with the patient, family, and interdisciplinary healthcare team, when possible and appropriate.

- Ensures that outcomes are realistic and attainable within the patient's available resources, cultural influences, and present and potential capabilities.

- Documents expected outcomes as measurable goals.

ADDITIONAL COMPETENCIES FOR THE NEUROSCIENCE ADVANCED PRACTICE REGISTERED NURSE

The neuroscience advanced practice registered nurse:

- Identifies expected outcomes that incorporate scientific evidence and are achievable through implementation of evidence-based practices.

- Identifies expected outcomes that incorporate cost and clinical effectiveness, patient satisfaction, and continuity and consistency among providers.

- Identifies factors that hinder achievement of outcomes for patients, families, nurses, or systems.

- Differentiates outcomes that require care process interventions from those that require system-level interventions.

Standard 4. Planning

The neuroscience registered nurse develops a plan of care that prescribes strategies and alternatives to attain expected outcomes.

COMPETENCIES

The neuroscience registered nurse:

- Develops an individualized plan in partnership with the person, family, and others considering the person's characteristics or situation, including, but not limited to, neurologic status, values, beliefs, spiritual and health practices, preferences, choices, developmental level, coping style, culture and environment, and available technology.

- Establishes the plan priorities with the patient, family, and others as appropriate.

- Includes strategies in the plan that address each of the identified diagnoses or issues. These strategies may include, but are not limited to, strategies for promotion and restoration of health; prevention of illness, injury, and disease; alleviation of suffering; and supportive care for those who are dying.

- Includes strategies for health and wholeness across the lifespan.

- Provides for continuity in the plan.

- Incorporates an implementation pathway or timeline in the plan.

- Considers the economic impact of the plan on the patient, family, caregivers, or other affected parties.

- Integrates current scientific evidence, trends, and research in developing the plan of care.

- Utilizes the plan to provide direction to other members of the healthcare team.

- Defines the plan to reflect current statutes, rules and regulations, and standards.

- Modifies the plan according to the ongoing assessment of the patient's response and other outcome indicators.

- Explores suggested, potential, and alternative options to the plan of care with the patient in a safe time and place.

- Documents the plan in a manner that uses standardized language or recognized terminology.

ADDITIONAL COMPETENCIES FOR THE
NEUROSCIENCE ADVANCED PRACTICE REGISTERED NURSE

The neuroscience advanced practice registered nurse:

- Identifies assessment strategies, diagnostic strategies, and therapeutic interventions that reflect current evidence, including data, research, literature, and expert clinical knowledge.

- Selects or designs strategies to meet the multifaceted needs of complex patients.

- Includes a synthesis of the patient's values and beliefs regarding nursing and medical therapies in the plan.

- Leads the design and development of interprofessional processes to address the identified diagnosis or issue.

- Actively participates in the development and continuous improvement of systems that support the planning process.

Standard 5. Implementation

The neuroscience registered nurse implements the identified plan.

COMPETENCIES

The neuroscience registered nurse:

- Partners with the person, family, significant others, and caregivers as appropriate to implement the plan in a safe, realistic, and timely manner.

- Demonstrates caring behaviors toward patients, significant others, and groups of people receiving care.

- Utilizes technology to measure, record, and retrieve patient data; implement the nursing process; and enhance nursing practice.

- Utilizes evidence-based interventions and treatments specific to the diagnosis or problem.

- Provides holistic care that addresses the needs of diverse populations across the lifespan.

- Advocates for healthcare that is sensitive to the needs of patients, with particular emphasis on the needs of diverse populations.

- Applies appropriate knowledge of major health problems and cultural diversity in implementing the plan of care.

- Applies available healthcare technologies to maximize access and optimize outcomes for patients.

- Utilizes community resources and systems to implement the plan.

- Collaborates with healthcare providers from diverse backgrounds to implement and integrate the plan.

- Accommodates different styles of communication used by patients, families, and healthcare providers.

- Integrates traditional and complementary healthcare practices as appropriate.

- Implements the plan in a timely manner in accordance with patient safety goals.

- Promotes the patient's capacity for the optimal level of participation and problem-solving.

- Documents implementation and any modifications, including changes or omissions, of the identified plan.

ADDITIONAL COMPETENCIES FOR THE NEUROSCIENCE ADVANCED PRACTICE REGISTERED NURSE

The neuroscience advanced practice registered nurse:

- Facilitates utilization of systems, organizations, and community resources to implement the plan.

- Supports collaboration with nursing and other colleagues to implement the plan.

- Incorporates new knowledge and strategies to initiate change in nursing care practices if desired outcomes are not achieved.

- Assumes responsibility for safe and efficient implementation of the plan.

- Utilizes advanced communication skills to promote relationships between nurses and patients, to provide a context for open discussion of the patient's experiences, and to improve patient outcomes.

- Actively participates in the development and continuous improvement of systems that support implementation of the plan.

Standard 5A. Coordination of Care

The neuroscience registered nurse coordinates care delivery.

COMPETENCIES

The neuroscience registered nurse:

- Organizes the components of the plan.

- Manages a patient's care in a way that maximizes independence and quality of life.

- Assists the patient to identify options for alternative care.

- Communicates with the patient, family, and system during transitions in care.

- Advocates for the delivery of dignified and humane care by the inter-professional team.

- Documents the coordination of care.

ADDITIONAL COMPETENCIES FOR THE NEUROSCIENCE ADVANCED PRACTICE REGISTERED NURSE

The neuroscience advanced practice registered nurse:

- Provides leadership in the coordination of interprofessional health care for integrated delivery of patient care services.

- Synthesizes data and information to prescribe necessary system and community support measures, including modifications of surroundings.

Standard 5B. Health Teaching and Health Promotion

The neuroscience registered nurse employs strategies to promote health and a safe environment for the patient with actual or potential neurologic dysfunction.

COMPETENCIES

The neuroscience registered nurse:

- Provides health teaching that addresses such topics as healthy lifestyles, risk-reducing behaviors, developmental needs, activities of daily living, and preventive self-care.

- Uses health promotion and health teaching methods appropriate to the situation and the patient's values, beliefs, health practices, developmental level, learning needs, readiness and ability to learn, language preference, spirituality, culture, and socioeconomic status.

- Seeks opportunities for feedback and evaluation of the effectiveness of the strategies used.

- Engages technology, in addition to using patient alliances and advocacy groups, in health teaching and health promotion activities.

- Provides patients with information about intended effects and potential adverse effects of proposed therapies.

ADDITIONAL COMPETENCIES FOR THE
NEUROSCIENCE ADVANCED PRACTICE REGISTERED NURSE

The neuroscience advanced practice registered nurse:

- Synthesizes empirical evidence on risk behaviors, learning theories, behavioral change theories, motivational theories, epidemiology, and other related theories and frameworks when designing health education information and programs.

- Conducts personalized health teaching and counseling after considering comparative effectiveness research recommendations.

- Designs health information and patient education appropriate to the patient's developmental level, learning needs, readiness to learn, and cultural values and beliefs.

- Evaluates health information resources, such as the Internet, in the area of practice for accuracy, readability, and comprehensibility to help patients access quality health information.

- Provides anticipatory guidance to individuals, families, groups, and communities to promote health and prevent or reduce the risk of health problems.

Standard 5C. Consultation

The neuroscience advanced practice registered nurse provides consultation to influence the identified plan for the patient, enhance the abilities of others, and effect change.

COMPETENCIES

The neuroscience advanced practice registered nurse:

- Synthesizes clinical data, theoretical frameworks, and evidence when providing consultation.

- Facilitates the effectiveness of a consultation by involving the patients and stakeholders in decision-making and negotiation of role responsibilities.

- Communicates consultation recommendations.

Standard 5D. Prescriptive Authority and Treatment

The neuroscience advanced practice registered nurse uses prescriptive authority, procedures, referrals, treatments, and therapies in accordance with state and federal laws and regulations.

COMPETENCIES
The neuroscience advanced practice registered nurse:

- Prescribes evidence-based treatments, therapies, and procedures considering the patient's comprehensive healthcare needs.

- Prescribes pharmacologic agents according to a current knowledge of pharmacology and physiology.

- Prescribes specific pharmacologic agents or treatments based on clinical indicators, the patient's status and needs, and the results of diagnostic and laboratory tests.

- Evaluates therapeutic and potential adverse effects of pharmacologic and nonpharmacologic treatments.

- Provides patients with information about intended effects and potential adverse effects of proposed prescriptive therapies. Provides information about costs and alternative treatments and procedures, as appropriate.

- Evaluates and incorporates complementary and alternative therapy into education and practice.

Standard 6. Evaluation

The neuroscience registered nurse evaluates the progress toward attainment of expected outcomes.

COMPETENCIES

The neuroscience registered nurse:

- Conducts a systematic, ongoing, and criterion-based evaluation of the outcomes in relation to the structures and processes prescribed by the plan of care and the indicated timeline.

- Collaborates with the patient and others involved in the care or situation in the evaluation process.

- Evaluates, in partnership with the patient, the effectiveness of the planned strategies in relation to the patient's responses and attainment of the expected outcomes.

- Uses ongoing assessment data to revise the diagnoses, the outcomes, the plan, and the implementation as needed.

- Disseminates the results to the patient, family, and others involved, in accordance with federal and state regulations.

- Participates in assessing and assuring the responsible and appropriate use of interventions to minimize unwarranted or unwanted treatment and patient suffering.

- Documents results of the evaluation.

ADDITIONAL COMPETENCIES FOR THE
NEUROSCIENCE ADVANCED PRACTICE REGISTERED NURSE

The neuroscience advanced practice registered nurse:

- Incorporates advanced nursing knowledge, quality scientific indicators, and best available evidence into evaluative measures.

- Analyzes findings from evaluative measures to assess effectiveness of the plan in attaining outcomes and its effect on the patient, families, groups, communities, and institutions.

■ Revises the diagnoses, expected outcomes, plan of care, and interventions to address outcomes that have not been met or have been only partially met.

■ Evaluates the accuracy of the diagnosis and the effectiveness of the interventions and other variables in relation to the patient's attainment of expected outcomes.

■ Disseminates evaluation findings to patients, families, groups, communities, and institutions, as well as to other interprofessional healthcare team members, to improve overall quality, satisfaction, and safety of care.

■ Modifies the plan of care for the trajectory of treatment according to evaluation of response.

■ Uses the results of the evaluation to make or recommend process or structural changes, including policy, procedure, or protocol revision, as appropriate.

Standards of Professional Performance for Neuroscience Nursing

Standard 7. Ethics

The neuroscience registered nurse practices ethically.

COMPETENCIES

The neuroscience registered nurse:

- Uses *Code of Ethics for Nurses with Interpretive Statements* (ANA, 2001) to guide practice.

- Delivers care in a manner that preserves and protects patient autonomy, dignity, rights, values, and beliefs.

- Recognizes the centrality of the patient and family as core members of any healthcare team.

- Upholds patient confidentiality within legal and regulatory parameters.

- Assists patients in self-determination and informed decision-making.

- Maintains a therapeutic and professional patient–nurse relationship within appropriate professional role boundaries.

- Identifies clinical situations in which ethical issues may develop.

- Contributes to resolving ethical issues involving patients, colleagues, community groups, systems, and other stakeholders.

- Takes appropriate action regarding instances of illegal, unethical, or inappropriate behavior that can endanger or jeopardize the best interests of the patient or situation.

- Questions healthcare practices when necessary for safety and quality improvement.

- Advocates for equitable patient care.

- Integrates caring, kindness, and respect into nursing practice.

- Participates in interprofessional teams that address ethical risks, benefits, and outcomes.

ADDITIONAL COMPETENCIES FOR THE NEUROSCIENCE ADVANCED PRACTICE REGISTERED NURSE

The neuroscience advanced practice registered nurse:

- Provides information on the risks, benefits, and outcomes of and alternatives to healthcare regimens to allow informed decision-making by the patient, including informed consent and informed refusal.

- Partners with interprofessional team members to address ethical risks, benefits, and outcomes of policies, programs, and services.

- Consults with others to resolve ethical issues of students, colleagues, or systems.

- Advocates for patient rights, an optimal care environment, access to care, and improved quality of care.

Standard 8. Education

The neuroscience registered nurse attains knowledge and competence that reflect current nursing practice.

COMPETENCIES

The neuroscience registered nurse:

- Participates in ongoing educational activities related to appropriate knowledge bases and professional issues.

- Demonstrates a commitment to lifelong learning through self-reflection and inquiry to address learning and personal growth needs.

- Seeks experiences that reflect current practice to maintain knowledge, skills, abilities, and judgment in clinical practice or role performance.

- Acquires knowledge and skills appropriate to the role, population, specialty, setting, role, or situation.

- Seeks formal and independent learning experiences to develop and maintain clinical and professional skills and knowledge.

- Identifies learning needs based on nursing knowledge, the various roles the nurse may assume, and the changing needs of the population.

- Participates in formal or informal consultations to address issues in nursing practice as an application of education and knowledge base.

- Shares educational findings, experiences, and ideas with peers.

- Contributes to a work environment conducive to the education of healthcare professionals.

- Maintains professional records that provide evidence of competence and lifelong learning.

- Seeks to obtain or maintain neuroscience nursing certification.

ADDITIONAL COMPETENCIES FOR THE
NEUROSCIENCE ADVANCED PRACTICE REGISTERED NURSE

The neuroscience advanced practice registered nurse:

- Uses current healthcare research findings and other evidence to expand clinical knowledge, skills, abilities, and judgment; to enhance role performance; and to increase knowledge of professional issues.

Standard 9. Evidence-Based Practice and Research

The neuroscience registered nurse integrates evidence and research findings into practice.

COMPETENCIES

The neuroscience registered nurse:

- Utilizes current evidence-based nursing knowledge, including research findings, to guide practice.

- Incorporates evidence when initiating changes in nursing practice.

- Participates, as appropriate to education level and position, in the formulation of evidence-based practice through research.

- Shares research findings with colleagues and peers.

ADDITIONAL COMPETENCIES FOR THE
NEUROSCIENCE ADVANCED PRACTICE REGISTERED NURSE

The neuroscience advanced practice registered nurse:

- Critically appraises research for practice.

- Utilizes research to enhance the environment of care and improve patient outcomes.

- Utilizes research skills in problem evaluation.

- Contributes to nursing knowledge by conducting or synthesizing research and other evidence that discovers, examines, and evaluates current practice, knowledge, theories, criteria, and creative approaches to improve healthcare outcomes.

- Promotes a climate of research and clinical inquiry.

- Disseminates research findings through activities such as presentations, publications, consultation, and journal clubs.

Standard 10. Quality of Practice

The neuroscience registered nurse contributes to quality nursing practice.

COMPETENCIES

The neuroscience registered nurse:

- Demonstrates quality by documenting the application of the nursing process in a responsible, accountable, and ethical manner.

- Uses creativity and innovation to enhance nursing care.

- Participates in quality improvement. Activities may include:

  - Identifying aspects of practice important for quality monitoring.

  - Using indicators to monitor quality, safety, and effectiveness of nursing practice.

  - Collecting data to monitor quality and effectiveness of nursing practice.

  - Analyzing quality data to identify opportunities for improving nursing practice.

  - Formulating recommendations to improve nursing practice or outcomes.

  - Implementing activities to enhance the quality of nursing practice.

  - Developing, implementing, and/or evaluating policies, procedures, and guidelines to improve the quality of practice.

  - Participating on and/or leading interprofessional teams to evaluate clinical care or health services.

  - Participating in and/or leading efforts to minimize costs and unnecessary duplication.

  - Identifying problems that occur in day-to-day work routines in order to correct process inefficiencies.

  - Analyzing factors related to quality, safety, and effectiveness.

- Analyzing organizational systems for barriers to quality patient outcomes.

- Implementing processes to remove or weaken barriers within organizational systems.

ADDITIONAL COMPETENCIES FOR THE
NEUROSCIENCE ADVANCED PRACTICE REGISTERED NURSE

The neuroscience advanced practice registered nurse:

- Provides leadership in the design and implementation of quality improvements.

- Designs innovations to effect change in practice and improve health outcomes.

- Evaluates the practice environment and quality of nursing care rendered in relation to existing evidence.

- Identifies opportunities for the generation and use of research and evidence.

- Obtains and maintains professional certification if it is available in the area of expertise.

- Uses the results of quality improvement activities to initiate changes in nursing practice throughout the healthcare delivery system.

Standard 11. Communication

The neuroscience registered nurse communicates effectively in a variety of formats in all areas of practice.

COMPETENCIES

The neuroscience registered nurse:

- Assesses communication format preferences of patients, families, and colleagues.

- Assesses her or his own communication skills in encounters with patients, families, and colleagues.

- Seeks continuous improvement of her or his own communication and conflict resolution skills.

- Conveys information to patients, families, the interprofessional team, and others in communication formats that promote accuracy.

- Questions the rationale supporting care processes and decisions when they do not appear to be in the best interest of the patient.

- Discloses observations or concerns related to hazards and errors in care or the practice environment to the appropriate level.

- Maintains communication with other providers to minimize risks associated with transfers and transition in care delivery.

- Contributes her or his own professional perspective in discussions with the interprofessional team.

Standard 12. Leadership

The neuroscience registered nurse demonstrates leadership in the professional practice setting and the profession.

COMPETENCIES

The neuroscience registered nurse:

- Oversees the nursing care given by others while retaining accountability for the quality of care given to the patient.

- Abides by the vision, the associated goals, and the plan to implement and measure progress of an individual patient or progress within the context of the healthcare organization.

- Demonstrates a commitment to continuous, lifelong learning and education for self and others.

- Mentors colleagues for the advancement of nursing practice, the profession, and quality health care.

- Treats colleagues with respect, trust, and dignity.

- Develops communication and conflict resolution skills.

- Participates in professional organizations.

- Communicates effectively with the patient and colleagues.

- Seeks ways to advance nursing autonomy and accountability.

- Participates in efforts to influence healthcare policy involving patients and the profession.

ADDITIONAL COMPETENCIES FOR THE
NEUROSCIENCE ADVANCED PRACTICE REGISTERED NURSE

The neuroscience advanced practice registered nurse:

- Influences decision-making bodies to improve the professional practice environment and patient outcomes.

- Provides direction to enhance the effectiveness of the interprofessional team.

■ Promotes advanced practice nursing and role development by interpreting its role for patients, families, and others.

■ Models expert practice to interprofessional team members and patients.

■ Mentors colleagues in the acquisition of clinical knowledge, skills, abilities, and judgment.

Standard 13. Collaboration

The neuroscience registered nurse collaborates with the patient, family, and others in the conduct of nursing practice.

COMPETENCIES

The neuroscience registered nurse:

- Partners with others to effect change and enhance positive outcomes by sharing knowledge of the patient and/or situation.

- Communicates with the patient, family, and healthcare providers regarding patient care and the nurse's role in the provision of that care.

- Promotes conflict management and resolution.

- Participates in building consensus or resolving conflict in the context of patient care.

- Applies group process and negotiation techniques with patients and colleagues.

- Adheres to standards and applicable codes of conduct that govern behavior among peers and colleagues to create a work environment that promotes cooperation, respect, and trust.

- Cooperates in creating a documented plan focused on outcomes and decisions related to care and delivery of services that indicates communication with patients, families, and others.

- Engages in teamwork and team-building processes.

ADDITIONAL COMPETENCIES FOR THE
NEUROSCIENCE ADVANCED PRACTICE REGISTERED NURSE

The neuroscience advanced practice registered nurse:

- Partners with other professions to enhance patient outcomes through interprofessional activities, including education, consultation, management, technological development, or research opportunities.

- Invites the contribution of the patient, family, and team members in order to achieve optimal outcomes.

- Leads in establishing, improving, and sustaining collaborative relationships to achieve safe, quality patient care.

- Documents plan-of-care communications, rationales for plan-of-care changes, and collaborative discussions to improve patient outcomes.

Standard 14. Professional Practice Evaluation

The neuroscience registered nurse evaluates her or his own nursing practice in relation to professional practice standards and guidelines, relevant statutes, rules, and regulations.

COMPETENCIES

The neuroscience registered nurse:

- Provides age-appropriate and developmentally appropriate care in a culturally and ethnically sensitive manner.

- Engages in performance appraisal on a regular basis, seeking constructive feedback regarding her or his own practice according to professional standards, and identifying areas of strength as well as areas where professional development would be beneficial.

- Obtains informal feedback regarding her or his own practice from patients, peers, professional colleagues, and others.

- Participates in peer review as appropriate.

- Takes action to achieve goals identified during the evaluation process.

- Provides the evidence for practice decisions and actions as part of the informal and formal evaluation processes.

- Interacts with peers and colleagues to enhance her or his own professional nursing practice or role performance.

- Provides peers with formal or informal constructive feedback regarding their practice or role performance.

ADDITIONAL COMPETENCIES FOR THE
NEUROSCIENCE ADVANCED PRACTICE REGISTERED NURSE

The neuroscience advanced practice registered nurse:

- Engages in a formal process of seeking feedback regarding her or his practice from peers, professional colleagues, patients, and others.

- Incorporates practice performance reviews and findings from peers, professional colleagues, patients, and others as appropriate into practice.

Standard 15. Resource Utilization

The neuroscience registered nurse utilizes appropriate resources to plan and provide nursing services that are safe, effective and financially responsible.

COMPETENCIES

The neuroscience registered nurse:

- Assesses individual patient care needs and resources available to achieve desired outcomes.

- Identifies patient care needs, potential for harm, complexity of the task, and desired outcome when considering resource allocation.

- Delegates elements of care to appropriate healthcare workers in accordance with any applicable legal or policy parameters or principles.

- Identifies the evidence when evaluating resources.

- Advocates for resources, including technology, that enhance nursing practice.

- Modifies practice when necessary to promote positive interaction between patients, care providers, and technology.

- Assists the patient and family in identifying and securing appropriate services to address needs across the healthcare continuum.

- Assists the patient and family in factoring costs, risks, and benefits in decisions about treatment and care.

ADDITIONAL COMPETENCIES FOR THE NEUROSCIENCE ADVANCED PRACTICE REGISTERED NURSE

The neuroscience advanced practice registered nurse:

- Utilizes organizational and community resources to formulate inter-professional plans of care.

- Formulates innovative solutions for patient care problems that utilize resources effectively and maintain quality.

- Designs evaluation strategies that demonstrate cost-effectiveness, cost benefit, and efficiency factors associated with nursing practice.

- Serves as an expert resource to influence healthcare policy.

Standard 16. Environmental Health

The neuroscience registered nurse practices in an environmentally safe and healthy manner.

COMPETENCIES

The neuroscience registered nurse:

- Attains knowledge of environmental health concepts, such as implementation of environmental health strategies.

- Promotes a practice environment that reduces environmental health risks for workers and patients.

- Assesses the practice environment for factors that threaten health, such as sound, odor, noise, and light.

- Advocates for the judicious and appropriate use of products in health care.

- Communicates environmental health risks and exposure reduction strategies to patients, families, colleagues, and communities.

- Utilizes scientific evidence to determine if a product or treatment is an environmental threat.

- Participates in strategies to promote healthy communities.

ADDITIONAL COMPETENCIES FOR THE
NEUROSCIENCE ADVANCED PRACTICE REGISTERED NURSE

The neuroscience advanced practice registered nurse:

- Creates partnerships that promote sustainable environmental health policies and conditions.

- Analyzes the impact of social, political, and economic influences on the environment and human health exposures.

- Critically evaluates the manner in which environmental health issues are presented by the popular media.

- Advocates for implementation of environmental principles for nursing practice.

- Supports nurses in advocating for and implementing environmental principles in nursing practice.

Glossary

Advanced practice registered nurse (APRN). A nurse who has completed an accredited graduate-level education that prepares her or him for the role of certified nurse practitioner, certified registered nurse anesthetist, certified nurse midwife, or clinical nurse specialist; has passed a national certification examination that measures the APRN role and population-focused competencies; maintains continued competence as evidenced by recertification; and is licensed to practice as an APRN.

Assessment. The first step of the nursing process, in which data about the patient are systematically and comprehensively collected.

Competence. The state of having the knowledge, judgment, skills, energy, experience, and motivation required to respond safely, effectively, and appropriately to nursing performance expectations and professional responsibilities (Roach, 2002). Competence is definable and measurable, and can be evaluated. An individual who demonstrates competence is performing successfully at an expected level.

Competency. An expected level of performance that integrates knowledge, skills, abilities, and judgment, based on established scientific knowledge and expectations for nursing practice. Competency statements are specific, measurable elements that interpret, explain, and facilitate practical use of the standard.

Diagnosis. The second step of the nursing process, in which the analysis of assessed data results in a clinical judgment expressed as a statement of the patient's response to actual or potential health needs or conditions. The diagnosis provides the basis for determining a plan to achieve expected outcomes.

Evaluation. The sixth and final step of the nursing process, in which the nurse systematically and continuously appraises progress toward attainment of outcomes; measurable elements that interpret, explain, and facilitate practical use of the standard.

Formal learning. A means of integrating knowledge, skills, abilities, and judgment, which most often occurs in structured, academic, and professional development environments.

Health care. The prevention, treatment, and management of illness; the preservation of mental and physical well-being; and the promotion of health through the services offered by a healthcare provider or health professional.

Healthcare provider. A person licensed to provide direct care to individuals, including diagnosis and treatment of acute and chronic health problems.

Healthy work environment. An employment atmosphere characterized by optimal physical, psychological, economic, and political conditions conducive to optimal productivity, including worker and patient safety, employer support and encouragement, absence of undue stress, and reasonable and sustainable staffing conditions and caseloads.

Implementation. The fifth step of the nursing process, in which the nurse acts to bring about the plan. In the standards of practice, the process of implementation has several components: include coordination of care; health teaching and health promotion; consultation; and, for the APRN, prescriptive authority and treatment.

Informal learning. A means of integrating knowledge, skills, abilities, and judgment into experiential insights gained in work, community, home, and other settings.

Interprofessional. Reliant on the overlapping knowledge, skills, and abilities of each professional team member. This can drive synergistic effects by which outcomes are enhanced and become more comprehensive than a simple aggregation of the individual efforts of the team members.

Judgment. A characteristic of nursing competence that includes critical thinking, problem solving, ethical reasoning, and decision-making.

Knowledge. A characteristic of nursing competence that encompasses thinking; understanding of science and humanities; professional standards of practice; and insights gained from practical experiences, personal capabilities, and leadership performance.

Liaison. A person whose function it is to maintain communication between or among individuals and an organization, parts of an organization, or between two or more organizations acting together for a common purpose.

Multidisciplinary team. A team of school or community professionals with a variety of skills, abilities, and disciplinary backgrounds who work together for a common purpose.

Nursing process. A circular, continuous, and dynamic critical thinking process comprised of six steps and that is patient-centered, interpersonal, collaborative, and universally applicable. The six steps are assessment, diagnosis, outcomes identification, planning, implementation, and evaluation. The nursing process encompasses all significant actions taken by registered nurses and forms the foundation of the neuroscience nurse's decision-making.

Outcomes identification. The third step of the nursing process, wherein measurable, expected, realistic, and attainable expectations for the patient are stipulated.

Planning. The fourth step of the nursing process, in which the nurse formulates a comprehensive outline of care to be implemented for attainment of specific measurable outcomes.

Population. Includes aggregates, persons with identified similarities, and communities.

Skills. A characteristic of nursing competence that includes psychomotor, communication, interpersonal, and diagnostic abilities.

Standards. Authoritative statements of the duties that all registered nurses, regardless of role, population, or specialty, are expected to perform.

System. Any group of interacting, interrelated, or interdependent elements forming a complex whole.

References

American Association of Critical Care Nurses (AACN). (2005). *AACN standards for establishing and maintaining healthy work environments.* Mission Viejo, CA: AACN.

American Nurses Association (ANA). (2001). *Code of ethics for nurses with interpretive statements.* Washington, DC: Nursesbooks.org.

American Nurses Association (ANA). (2008). *Professional role competence* (Position Statement). Silver Spring, MD: Author.

American Nurses Association (ANA). (2010a). *Nursing: Scope and standards of practice* (2nd ed.). Silver Spring, MD: Nursesbooks.org.

American Nurses Association (ANA). (2010b). *Nursing's social policy statement: The essence of the profession.* Silver Spring, MD: Nursesbooks.org.

American Nurses Credentialing Center (ANCC). (2008). *A new model for ANCC's Magnet Recognition Program*®. Silver Spring, MD: Author.

APRN Joint Dialogue Group (JDG). (2008). *Consensus model for APRN regulation: Licensure, accreditation, certification, and education.* Retrieved from http://www.nursingworld.org/ConsensusModelforAPRN

Bader, M. K., & Littlejohns, L. R (Eds.). (2010). *AANN core curriculum for neuroscience nursing* (5th ed.). Glenview, IL: American Association of Neuroscience Nurses.

Diorio, C., Hinkle, J., Stuifbergen, A., Algase, D., Amidei, C., et al. (2011). Updated research priorities for neuroscience nursing. *Journal of Neuroscience Nursing, 43*(3), 149–155.

Fowler, M. D. M. (Ed.). (2008). *Guide to the code of ethics for nurses: Interpretation and application.* Silver Spring, MD: Nursesbooks.org.

Gallagher-Lepak, S., & Kubsch, S. (2009). Transpersonal caring: A nursing practice guideline. *Holistic Nursing Practice, 23*(3), 171–182.

Hagerty, B. M., Lynch-Sauer, J., Patusky, K. L., & Bouwsema, M. (1993). An emerging theory of human relatedness. *Image: Journal of Nursing Scholarship, 25*(4), 291–296.

Holleman, J., Johnson, A., & Frim, D. (2010). The impact of a "resident replacement" nurse practitioner on an academic pediatric neurosurgical service. *Pediatric Neurosurgery, 46*(3), 177–181.

Institute of Medicine (IOM). (2004). *Patient safety: Achieving a new standard for care.* Washington, DC: Author.

Institute of Medicine. (2009). "Technology-enabled nursing" and "Reactions and questions," in *Forum on the future of nursing: Acute care* (ch. 4, Technology, pp. 28–33). Washington, DC: National Academies Press. Retrieved from http://www.nap.edu/catalog.php?record_id=12855

Kane, R. L., Shamilyan, T., Mueller, C., Duval, S., & Wilt, T. J. (2007). *Nurse staffing and quality of patient care.* Rockville, MD: Agency for Healthcare Research and Quality.

Mills, N., Bachmann, M. O., Campbell, R., Hine, I., & McGowan, M. (1999). Effect of a primary care based epilepsy specialist nurse service on quality of care from the patients' perspective: Results at two-years follow-up. *Seizure, 8*(5), 291–296.

Roach, M. S. (2002). *Caring, the human mode of being: A blueprint for the health professions* (2nd ed.). Ottawa, Ontario, Canada: CHA Press (Presses de l'ACS).

Stewart-Amidei, C., & Kunkel, J. A. (Eds.). (2000). *AANN's neuroscience nursing: Human responses to neurologic dysfunction* (2nd ed). Philadelphia: Saunders.

Stewart-Amidei, C., Villanueva, N., Schwartz, R. R., Delemos, C., West, T., Tocco, S., et al. (2010). American Association of Neuroscience Nurses scope and standards of practice for neuroscience advanced practice nurses. *Journal of Neuroscience Nursing, 42*(3), E1–E8.

Styles, M. M., Schumann, M. J., Bickford, C., & White, K. M. (2008). *Specialization and credentialing in nursing revisited.* Silver Spring, MD: Nursesbooks.org.

Unruh, L. (2008). Nurse staffing and patient, nurse and financial outcomes. *American Journal of Nursing, 108*(1), 62–71.

Villanueva, N., Blank-Reid, C., Stewart-Amidei, C., Cartwright, C., Haymore, J., & Jones, R. W. (2008). The role of the advanced practice nurse in neuroscience nursing. *Journal of Neuroscience Nursing, 40*(2), 119–124.

Watson, J. (2008). Social justice and human caring: A model of caring science as a hopeful paradigm for moral justice for humanity. *Creative Nursing, 14*(2), 54–61.

Webb, D. (2000). Scope of neuroscience nursing. In C. Stewart-Amidei & J. A. Kunkel (Eds.), *AANN's neuroscience nursing: Human responses to neurologic dysfunction* (2nd ed., pp. 3–11). Philadelphia: Saunders.

Yeager, S., Shaw, K. D., Casavant, J., & Burns, S. M. (2006). An acute care nurse practitioner model of care for neurosurgical patients. *Critical Care Nurse 26*(6), 57–64.

Appendix A.

Scope and Standards of Neuroscience Nursing Practice (2002)

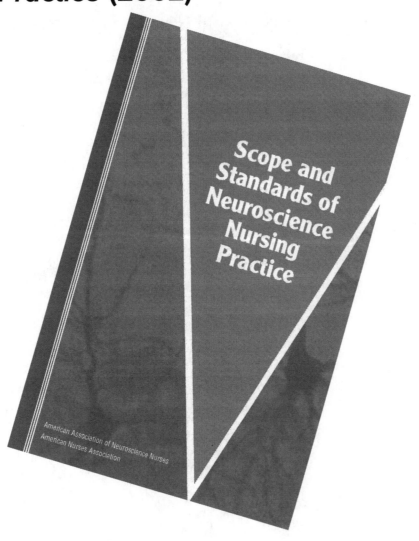

Scope and Standards of Neuroscience Nursing Practice

American Association of Neuroscience Nurses
American Nurses Association

The content in this appendix is not current and is of historical significance only.

Scope and Standards
of
Neuroscience Nursing Practice

American Association of Neuroscience Nurses

American Nurses Association

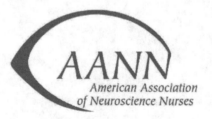

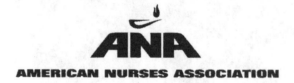

Washington, D.C.

The content in this appendix is not current and is of historical significance only.

ACKNOWLEDGMENTS

The task force that created this document gratefully acknowledges the work of previous task forces in 1977, 1986, 1993, and 2001 that initiated the original documents on Neuroscience Nursing Practice.

The American Association of Neuroscience Nurses (AANN) Scope and Standards Practice Task Force developed this document.

Task Force Members

Susan Bell, RN, MS, CNRN, CNP, Task Force Chairperson

Laura McIlvoy, RN, MSN, CCRN, CNRN

Janice L. Hinkle, RN, PhD, CNRN

Susan Fowler, RN, PhD, CCRN, CNRN, CS

Chris Stewart-Amidei, RN, MSN, CNRN

Janette Yanko, RN, MN, CNRN

Tess Sierzant, MSN, RN, CNRN

Susan Young, MN

AANN Board of Director's Liaison
Michelle VanDemark

AANN Staff Liaison
Louise S. Miller, MA

American Nurses Association (ANA) Staff
Carol Bickford, MS, RN, C
Yvonne Humes, BBA

Special thanks to Karen Ballard, MA, RN for her review of the early drafts of this document.

The content in this appendix is not current and is of historical significance only.

CONTENTS

PREFACE

Neuroscience nursing was formally recognized as a specialty in 1968 with the formation of the American Association of Neurosurgical Nurses (AANN). In 1985, this name was changed to the American Association of Neuroscience Nurses to reflect the practice diversity of its members.

A statement of neuroscience nursing's scope of practice was first completed in 1986 by the AANN Nursing Practice Committee. This document served to describe the parameters of nursing practice for the specialty, identify the population served and practice settings, and distinguish qualifications of nurses in the specialty and the type of care rendered to patients. This description is useful to the neuroscience nurse in defining goals and to the public for clarifying expectations.

Revised in 1993, the next scope of practice statement addressed the expanded options for neuroscience nursing in the 1990s. This revision in 2002 reflects evolving practice in the new century. The borders of nursing practice have grown in recent years with potential for continued change as health care reforms take shape. A renewed emphasis is also being placed on the care of patients across the lifespan and a spectrum of health states rather than a focus on episodes of illness. This new statement's intent is to describe neuroscience nursing practice in terms broad enough to include all the possibilities, yet specific enough to remain useful.

The content in this appendix is not current and is of historical significance only.

NEUROSCIENCE NURSING SCOPE OF PRACTICE

Neuroscience nursing is a unique area within the nursing discipline, which specializes in the care of individuals who have biological, psychological, social, and spiritual alterations due to nervous system dysfunction. This encompasses all levels of human existence, from basic bodily functions to advanced processes of the human mind. Neuroscience nursing care is provided across the lifespan, from birth through death. Major categories of disease that produce alterations of concern to neuroscience nurses include degenerative diseases, tumors of the nervous system, neuromuscular diseases, traumatic injury to the nervous system, cerebrovascular disease, seizures, pain, diseases of the spine, movement disorders, and developmental problems of the nervous system. Potential recipients of neuroscience nursing care are individuals with nervous system dysfunction, their families and significant others, and the society in which they live. Neuroscience nursing also includes prevention of nervous system dysfunction through education, health promotion, and research.

Practice Characteristics

Neuroscience nurses identify and treat human responses to actual or potential health problems related to phenomena affected by nervous system dysfunction. Specific phenomena that form the framework for neuroscience nursing practice include:

- *Consciousness and Cognition*—The awareness of and interaction with the surrounding environment as well as the higher thought processes; alterations include problems such as coma, memory impairment, and seizures.

- *Communication*—The language interaction with others; alterations include language impairments secondary to the aphasias or dysarthria.

- *Mobility*—The ability to move freely within the environment; alterations include various forms of paralysis

- *Affiliative Relationships*—The ability to form and maintain social support relationships; alterations include social isolation and role changes secondary to nervous system disease.

- *Rest and Sleep*—Phenomena necessary for restorative function; alterations include the spectrum of sleep disorders.

- *Sensation*—The ability to sense and distinguish internal and external stimuli; alterations include decreased sensation and pain.

- *Elimination*—Bodily excretion of waste products; alterations include bowel and bladder dysfunction secondary to nervous system disease.

- *Sexuality*—The ability to interact and maintain a sexual relationship; alterations include sexual dysfunction secondary to nervous system disease.

- *Self-care*—The ability to provide for one's basic needs; alterations include the inability to care for one's self.

- *Integrated Regulation*—The interrelationship between the nervous system and other body systems; alterations include loss of regulatory control.

Neuroscience nurses use the nursing process to deliver care (assessment, diagnosis, outcome identification and planning, implementation, evaluation). Although this begins with assessment, specific attention is focused on neurological assessment. Data gathered from the neurological assessment are used to plan and implement nursing interventions specific to the patient's neurologic dysfunction. Interventions may support bodily functions and promote healing and recovery of the acutely ill; enhance adaptation to persistent neurologic deficits for the chronically ill; facilitate patient, family and significant other coping; and teach patients, families, and significant others about disease processes, adaptation techniques, and therapies. The neuroscience nurse evaluates the outcomes of nursing care on an ongoing basis, and revises the plan as necessary. Further, review and application of related clinical relevant and evidenced-based research results in the promotion of creative therapeutic nursing interventions and improved patient outcomes. Care is guided by the Neuroscience Nursing Standards of Practice, and ethical principles are applied in any care rendered.

Practice Environment, Education, Certification, and Roles

The neuroscience nurse may practice in a variety of settings. Most care is delivered in inpatient or outpatient settings, but may be delivered in the home or community. Care areas may include pre-hospital, emergency, intensive, acute, ambulatory or chronic care, the operating room, and rehabilitation setting among others. Nurses work with either a broad range of patients with neurologic dysfunction and their families and significant others, or with a specific population of patients such as those with stroke, head injury, spinal cord injury, epilepsy, or brain tumors to name a few.

Graduation from a basic nursing education program and registered nurse licensure are required for entry into the neuroscience nursing field. An appropriate orientation program supports initial practice. Continuing education activities and involvement in the specialty's professional organization support ongoing practice. Advanced practice in neuroscience nursing requires additional formal education, including knowledge of nursing theory; the applied, social, and behavioral sciences; and advanced nursing assessment and therapeutics.

Professionalism is demonstrated by assuming accountability for maintaining excellence in practice through self-motivated ventures, as well as collaborative efforts with other nursing colleagues, organizations, and intraprofessional associates. Participation in the specialty's certification process further identifies the nurse's expertise in neuroscience nursing. Nurses who have worked in neuroscience nursing for at least two years may choose to test their proficiency in neuroscience nursing to become a Certified Neuroscience Registered Nurse (CNRN). Ongoing certification may be retained either through continuing education or retesting.

Beyond direct delivery of care, the neuroscience nurse may practice in a variety of roles, such as educator, administrator, researcher, consultant, and clinical expert. Each role is based upon specific clinical expertise, and education. Basic nursing role titles may include staff nurse with varying degrees of advancement. Advanced practice role titles may include clinical nurse specialist or nurse practitioner.

In all of the identified settings, levels of practice, and roles, the primary intent is to care for, support, teach, and serve as an advocate for the patient. The goal of all intervention in neuroscience nursing practice is consistent with and flows from that of the entire nursing profession: to

The content in this appendix is not current and is of historical significance only.

provide the highest quality of care to patients and achieve a state of wellness consistent with the quality of life desired by the patient, which may include a peaceful and dignified death.

Future Considerations

The evolving nature of neuroscience nursing is a reflection of techno-logical advances, greater scientific understanding, and a rapidly grow-ing research base. Nursing has moved from an era of needing only to provide good, safe, physical care to the patient with severe neurologic dysfunction to the present era of explicit incorporation of science and research into care. An example of this is the early treatment of stroke. Ten years ago, stroke care consisted of supportive and rehabilitative care only. It is now possible to reverse stroke deficits with early inter-vention, and neuroscience nurses play a key role in this process.

Neuroscience nurses are increasingly involved in research activities, not just as consumers, but as independent or collaborative researchers. Advances in the various branches of science, such as neurogenetics, are rapidly changing the face of neuroscience nursing practice. Genet-ics may broaden treatment options, and nurses must not only be aware of the clinical implications of this, but the ethical implications as well. Complementary medicine and alternative therapies are further expand-ing the health care options, challenging neuroscience nurses to keep abreast of those developments and guide their patients in their use.

A major impact on the scope of practice in neuroscience nursing is the changing health care delivery system. Societal, economic, and political pressures are driving the development of less costly means to meet the health care needs of the public. One way neuroscience nurses can be intimately involved in this process is by using nurse specialists to deliver care. Advanced practice nurses, with their expanded knowledge base and expertise, can provide high quality care in a more cost-effective manner. An example of this might be a nurse-managed seizure clinic. These advanced practice nurses can also function as consultants to other nurses and other health care team members. Collaboration, along with effective use of resources, cost-containment, increased participation by recipients of care, timely achievement of goals, and continuity of care are concepts critical to the future of neuroscience nursing as well as other health care systems.

The changing health care market will also have an impact on the practice of neuroscience nursing. As the population of the United States ages, chronic illness will predominate, and a paradigm shift from acute to chronic illness will be necessary. Neuroscience nurses are challenged to redirect their practice, and educators are challenged to meet the demand for practitioners. The focus of health care providers is evolving to address prevention and problem management across the lifespan, rather than focusing on episodic care alone. Indeed, a major shift from inpatient to outpatient care settings is occurring. More expanded roles in community-based programs are likely. Nursing interactions are moving beyond the traditional settings into novel areas such as industry, legal practice, insurance, and social service areas.

As these changes evolve, neuroscience nurses will be at the forefront. Critical to the future of neuroscience nursing is the ability to recruit an adequate number of nurses to the specialty, as well as retain those who are currently practicing. But, the major responsibility of neuroscience nursing will remain the realm of human responses to actual or potential health problems secondary to nervous system dysfunction.

The content in this appendix is not current and is of historical significance only.

STANDARDS OF NEUROSCIENCE NURSING PRACTICE

Definition and Role of Standards

> Standards are authoritative statements by which the nursing profession describes the responsibilities for which its practitioners are accountable. Consequently, standards reflect the values and priorities of the profession. Standards provide direction for professional nursing practice and a framework for the evaluation of nursing practice. Written in measurable terms, standards also define the nursing profession's accountability to the public and the client outcomes for which nurses are responsible (ANA 1998, p. 1).

Guidelines, as distinguished from standards, "describe a process of patient care management which has the potential for improving the quality of clinical and consumer decision-making" (ANA, 1998, p. 5). *Guidelines* address the care of specific patient populations or phenomena, whereas *standards* provide a broad framework for practice. Standards generally remain stable over time, reflecting the philosophical values of the profession and current state of the art. Standards can be revised and updated to reflect changes in scientific knowledge and clinical practice within the specialty.

Development of Standards

"A professional nursing organization has a responsibility to its membership and to the public it serves to develop standards of practice" (ANA 1998, p. 1). This document sets forth standards of clinical practice for the specialty of neuroscience nursing and describes a competent level of professional performance common to all nurses engaged in the practice of neuroscience nursing, regardless of practice setting. These standards of neuroscience nursing practice consist of Standards of Care and Standards of Professional Performance.

The content in this appendix is not current and is of historical significance only.

Standards of Care

The six Standards of Care, as demonstrated by the nursing process, describe a competent level of nursing care and include assessment, diagnosis, outcome identification, planning, implementation, and evaluation. "The nursing process encompasses all significant actions taken by nurses in providing care to all clients, and forms the foundation of clinical decision-making" (ANA 1998, pp. 3–4). Several themes span across all areas of nursing practice and reflect nursing responsibilities for all patients. These themes include (ANA 1998, p. 4):

- providing age–appropriate and culturally and ethnically sensitive care
- maintaining a safe environment
- educating patients about healthy practices and treatment modalities
- assuring continuity of care
- coordinating the care across settings and among caregivers
- managing information
- communicating effectively.

Standards of Professional Performance

The eight Standards of Professional Performance describe a competent level of behavior in the professional role and include activities related to quality of care, performance appraisal, education, collegiality, ethics, collaboration, research, and resource utilization. "All nurses are expected to engage in professional role activities appropriate to their education and position. Ultimately, nurses are accountable to themselves, their patients, and their peers for their professional actions" (ANA 1998, p. 4).

The content in this appendix is not current and is of historical significance only.

Measurement Criteria

Measurement criteria are key indicators of competent practice that allow the standards to be measured. For the standards to be met, all criteria must be achieved.

The terms *appropriate, pertinent,* and *realistic* are used throughout this document. "The nurse will need to exercise judgement based on education and experience in determining what is appropriate, pertinent, or realistic. Further direction may be available from documents, such as guidelines for practice or agency standards, policies, procedures, and protocols" (ANA, 1998 p. 5).

The content in this appendix is not current and is of historical significance only.

STANDARDS OF CARE OF
NEUROSCIENCE NURSING PRACTICE

STANDARD I. ASSESSMENT
The neuroscience nurse collects health data.

Measurement Criteria

1. Data collection involves the patients, families, significant others, and other health care providers as appropriate.

2. The priority of data collection activities is determined by the patient's condition or needs.

3. Pertinent data are collected using appropriate assessment techniques and instruments using a variety of valid and reliable examinations, scales, tools, and equipment.

4. Relevant data are documented in a retrievable form.

5. The data collection process is systematic and ongoing.

6. The data collection process is comprehensive according to the patient's needs and system responses.

STANDARD II. DIAGNOSIS
The neuroscience nurse analyzes the assessment data in determining diagnoses.

Measurement Criteria

1. Diagnoses are derived from the assessment data.

2. Diagnoses are validated with the patient, family, significant other, and other health care providers, when possible and appropriate.

3. Diagnoses are documented in a manner that facilitates the determination of expected outcomes and plan of care.

The content in this appendix is not current and is of historical significance only.

STANDARD III. OUTCOME IDENTIFICATION
The neuroscience nurse identifies expected outcomes individualized to the patient.

Measurement Criteria

1. Outcomes are derived from the assessment and the diagnosis on an ongoing basis.

2. Outcomes are mutually formulated with the patient, family, and other heath care providers, when possible and appropriate.

3. Identified outcomes are consistent with current scientific evidence.

4. Outcomes are culturally appropriate and realistic in relation to the patient's present and potential capabilities.

5. Outcomes are attainable in relation to resources available to the patient.

6. Outcomes include a time estimate for attainment.

7. Outcomes provide direction for continuity of care.

8. Outcomes are documented as measurable short- or long-term goals.

STANDARD IV. PLANNING
The neuroscience nurse develops a plan of care that prescribes interventions to attain expected outcomes.

Measurement Criteria

1. The plan is individualized to the patient (e.g., age-appropriate, culturally sensitive) and the patient's neurological condition and potential.

2. The plan is developed with the patient, family, and other health care providers, as appropriate.

3. The plan reflects current state of the art of neuroscience nursing practice.

4. The plan proposes alternatives for continuity of care along the health care continuum.

5. The plan provides for continuity of care.

6. Priorities for care are established with the patient, family, and other health care providers.

7. The plan is documented.

8. The plan is communicated to the patient, family, and other health care providers.

9. The plan accommodates the changing nature of the patient and family's needs.

STANDARD V. IMPLEMENTATION
The neuroscience nurse implements the interventions identified in the plan of care.

Measurement Criteria

1. Interventions are consistent with the established plan of care.

2. Interventions are implemented in a safe, timely, and appropriate manner.

3. Interventions are documented.

4. Interventions are implemented in accordance with family, patient, significant other and caregiver knowledge.

5. Interventions are of the restorative, supportive, or promotive type.

6. Interventions unique to neuroscience nurses have been identified by several role delineation studies utilizing the Nursing Interventions Classification (NIC).

STANDARD VI. EVALUATION
The neuroscience nurse evaluates the patient's progress toward attainment of expected outcomes.

Measurement Criteria

1. Evaluation is systematic, ongoing, and criterion-based.

2. The patient, family, and other health care providers are involved in the evaluation process, as appropriate.

3. Ongoing assessment data are used to revise diagnoses, outcomes, and the plan of care as needed.

4. Revisions in diagnoses, outcomes and the plan of care are documented and communicated to the patient, family, and other health care providers.

5. The effectiveness of interventions is evaluated in relation to outcomes.

6. The patient's responses to interventions are documented.

The content in this appendix is not current and is of historical significance only.

STANDARDS OF PROFESSIONAL PERFORMANCE OF NEUROSCIENCE NURSING PRACTICE

STANDARD I. QUALITY OF CARE
The neuroscience nurse systematically evaluates the quality and effectiveness of nursing practice

Measurement Criteria

1. The neuroscience nurse participates in quality of care and continuous quality of care activities as appropriate to the nurses' education, experience, and position. Such activities may include:

   - identification of aspects of care important for quality monitoring

   - analysis of quality data to identify opportunities for improving care

   - development of policies, procedures, and practice guidelines to improve quality of care

   - identification of indicators used to monitor quality and effectiveness of nursing care

   - collection of data to monitor quality and effectiveness of nursing care

   - formulation of recommendations to improve nursing practice or patient outcomes

   - implementation of activities to enhance the quality of nursing practice

   - participation on interdisciplinary teams that evaluate clinical practice or health services

2. The neuroscience nurse uses the results of continuous quality of care activities to initiate changes in nursing practice.

3. The neuroscience nurse uses the results of continuous quality of care activities to initiate changes throughout the health care delivery system, as appropriate.

The content in this appendix is not current and is of historical significance only.

STANDARD II. PERFORMANCE APPRAISAL
The neuroscience nurse evaluates one's own practice in relation to professional practice standards and relevant statutes and regulations.

Measurement Criteria

1. The neuroscience nurse engages in performance appraisal on a regular basis, identifying areas of strength as well as areas where professional development would be beneficial.

2. The neuroscience nurse seeks constructive feedback regarding one's own practice.

3. The neuroscience nurse takes action to achieve goals identified during performance appraisal.

4. The neuroscience nurse participates in peer review as appropriate.

5. The neuroscience nurse's practice reflects knowledge of current professional practice standards, laws, and regulations.

STANDARD III. EDUCATION
The neuroscience nurse acquires and maintains current knowledge and competency in nursing practice.

Measurement Criteria

1. The neuroscience nurse participates in ongoing educational activities related to clinical and theoretical knowledge and professional issues.

2. The neuroscience nurse seeks experiences that reflect current clinical practice in order to maintain current clinical skills and competence.

3. The neuroscience nurse acquires knowledge and skills appropriate to the specialty and practice setting.

STANDARD IV. COLLEGIALITY

The neuroscience nurse interacts with, and contributes to the professional development of peers and other health care providers as colleagues.

Measurement Criteria

1. The neuroscience nurse shares knowledge and skills with colleagues.

2. The neuroscience nurse provides peers with constructive feedback regarding their practice.

3. The neuroscience nurse interacts with colleagues to enhance one's own professional nursing practice.

4. The neuroscience nurse contributes to an environment that is conducive to the clinical education of nursing students, other health care students, and other employees, as appropriate.

5. The neuroscience nurse contributes to a supportive and healthy work environment.

STANDARD V. ETHICS

The neuroscience nurse's decisions and actions on behalf of patients are determined in an ethical manner.

Measurement Criteria

1. The neuroscience nurse's practice is guided by the *Code of Ethics for Nurses with Interpretive Statements*.

2. The neuroscience nurse maintains patient confidentiality within legal and regulatory parameters.

3. The neuroscience nurse acts as a patient advocate and assists patients in developing skills so they can advocate for themselves.

4. The neuroscience nurse delivers care in a nonjudgmental and nondiscriminatory manner that is sensitive to patient diversity.

5. The neuroscience nurse delivers care in a manner that preserves patient autonomy, dignity, and rights.

6. The neuroscience nurse utilizes available resources in formulating ethical decisions.

The content in this appendix is not current and is of historical significance only.

STANDARD VI. COLLABORATION
The neuroscience nurse collaborates with the patient, family, and other health care providers in providing patient care.

Measurement Criteria

1. The neuroscience nurse communicates with the patient, family, and other health care providers regarding patient care and nursing's role in the provision of care.

2. The neuroscience nurse collaborates with the patient, family, and other health care providers in the formulation of overall goals and the plan of care and in decisions related to care and the delivery of services.

3. The neuroscience nurse consults with other health care providers for patient care, as needed.

4. The neuroscience nurse makes referrals, including provisions for continuity of care, as needed.

STANDARD VII. RESEARCH
The neuroscience nurse uses research findings in practice.

Measurement Criteria

1. The neuroscience nurse utilizes best available evidence, preferably research findings, to develop the plan of care and interventions.

2. The neuroscience nurse participates in research activities as appropriate to the nurse's education, experience, and position. Such activities may include:

   - identifying clinical problems suitable for nursing research

   - participating in data collection

   - participating in a unit, organization, or community research committee or program

   - sharing research activities with others

   - conducting research

   - critiquing research for application to practice

- using research findings in the development of policies, proce-dures, and practice guidelines for patient care
- using research findings to advance the state of nursing science in the care of neurological patients

STANDARD VIII. RESOURCE UTILIZATION
The neuroscience nurse considers factors related to safety, effectiveness, and cost in planning and delivering patient care.

Measurement Criteria

1. The neuroscience nurse evaluates factors related to safety, effec-tiveness, availability, and cost when choosing between two or more practice options that would result in the same expected patient outcome.

2. The neuroscience nurse assists the patient and family in identifying and securing appropriate and available services to address health-related needs.

3. The neuroscience nurse assigns or delegates tasks as defined by the state nurse practice acts and according to the knowledge and skills of the designated caregiver.

4. If the neuroscience nurse assigns or delegates tasks, it is based on the needs and condition of the patient, the potential for harm, the stability of the patient's condition, the complexity of the task, and the predictability of the outcome.

5. The neuroscience nurse assists the patient and family in becoming informed consumers about the cost, risks, and benefits of treatment and care.

The content in this appendix is not current and is of historical significance only.

REFERENCES

American Nurses Association. 1977. *Standards of Neurological and Neurosurgical Nursing Practice*. Kansas City, Mo.: American Nurses Association.

American Nurses Association. 1995. *Nursing's Social Policy Statement*. Washington, DC: American Nurses Publishing.

American Nurses Association & American Association of Neuroscience Nurses. 1985. *Neuroscience Nursing Practice: Process and Outcome Criteria for Selected Diagnosis*. Kansas City, Mo.: American Nurses Association.

American Nurses Association. 1985. *Code of Ethics for Nurses with Interpretive Statements*. Washington, DC: American Nurses Publishing.

American Nurses Association. 1998. *Standards of Clinical Nursing Practice* (2nd Edition). Washington, DC: American Nurses Publishing.

American Nurses Association. 1999. *Scope and Standards of Home Health Nursing Practice*. Washington, DC: American Nurses Publishing.

McCloskey, J.C., Bulechek, G.M., & Donahue, W. 1998. Nursing interventions core to specialty practice. *Nursing Outlook* 46: 67–76.

Quad Council of Public Health Organization & American Nurses Association. 1999. *Scope and Standards of Public Health Nursing Practice*. Washington, DC: American Nurses Publishing.

Stewart-Amidei, C., & Kunkel, J. 2001. AANN's *Neuroscience Nursing: Human Responses to Neurologic Dysfunction* (2nd Edition). Philadelphia: W.B. Saunders Company.

Appendix B.

Scope and Standards of Practice for Neuroscience Advanced Practice Nurses (2010)

The content in this appendix is not current and is of historical significance only.

American Association of Neuroscience Nurses Scope and Standards of Practice for Neuroscience Advanced Practice Nurses

Chris Stewart-Amidei, Nancy Villanueva, Rose Rossi Schwartz, Christi Delemos, Therese West, Susan Tocco, Cathy Cartwright, Rich Jones, Cindy Blank-Reid, Joseph Haymore

Background

Specialization in nursing arose as a way to enhance quality of care and improve access to care, in the face of increasing knowledge and technological advances. A nursing specialty is characterized by a unique body of knowledge and skill set, with nurses providing care focused on phenomena unique to the practice. *Neuroscience nursing* is a unique nursing discipline that addresses the needs of individuals with biopsychosocial alterations because of nervous system dysfunction (Webb, 2000). Recognition of neuroscience nursing as a practice specialty began in the 1960s and resulted in the formation of the American Association of Neurosurgical Nurses in 1968. To reflect the broader practice of its members, the association was renamed the American Association of Neuroscience Nurses in 1983.

Questions or comments about this article may be directed to Chris Stewart-Amidei, MSN RN CNRN CCRN FAAN at camidei@mail.ucf.edu. She is an instructor at University of Central Florida College of Nursing, Orlando, FL.

Nancy Villanueva, PhD CRNP BC CNRN, is a neurosurgical nurse practitioner at Penn State Milton S. Hershey Medical Center, Hershey, PA.

Rose Rossi Schwartz, PhD RN, is assistant professor of nursing, School of Nursing, Widener University, Chester, PA.

Christi Delemos, MS RN ACNP, is a nurse practitioner at University of California, Davis, CA.

Therese West, MSN RN APN-C, West Allehurst, NJ.

Susan Tocco, MSN RN CNRN CNS CCNS, is a neuroscience clinical nurse specialist at Orlando Regional Medical Center, Orlando, FL.

Cathy Cartwright, MSN RN PCNS, is a pediatric clinical nurse specialist in Neurosurgery, Children's Mercy Hospital, Kansas City, MO.

Rich Jones, BSN PNP CNRN RNFA, is a nurse practitioner in the office of Jeffrey Cone, MD, Amarillo, TX.

Cindy Blank-Reid, MSN RN CEN, is a trauma clinical nurse specialist at Temple University Medical Center, Philadelphia, PA.

Joseph Haymore, MS RN CNRN CCRN ACNP, is a neurosurgery and neurocritical care nurse practitioner at Neurocare Associates, Silver Spring, MD.

As neuroscience nursing evolved as a specialty, so did opportunities for advanced practice. The nursing shortage, the need to improve quality of care, restricted residency hours, and promotion of cost-effective care have led to increasing use of advanced practice nurses (APNs). The number of APNs in neuroscience nursing has grown in recent decades, reflecting the complexity and diversity of the field. Through education and certification, the neuroscience APN demonstrates basic competency in the role. Neuroscience APNs include clinical nurse specialists (CNSs) and nurse practitioners (NPs). Neuroscience APNs work in a variety of settings, demonstrate specific competencies unique to neuroscience nursing, and have a broad scope of responsibilities.

This document provides a framework for the neuroscience APN to practice, addressing the four requirements necessary for regulation of the advanced practice role: licensure, accreditation, certification, and education. Although neuroscience advanced practice nursing roles are defined, procedures and activities that may be performed are not defined because those are subject to individual collaborative practice as guided by state law and institutional or practice policy (Herrmann & Zabramski, 2005). There are many diverse statutes (state, federal, and community) and institutional guidelines that govern APN practice, and the Scope of Practice for Neuroscience Advanced Practice Nurses does not supersede those statutes or guidelines. For those APNs who are required to practice within a contractual agreement, protocols may be collaboratively developed that address specific responsibilities and expectations. The ability to perform specific clinical tasks is a multifaceted process involving APN competency, collaborative agreement with the physician or institution (if required), and state statutes. As practice evolves and statutes change, updates to this document may be necessary to reflect developments in the practice environment.

Definition and Scope of Practice

The American Association of Neuroscience Nurses defines the neuroscience APN as a registered nurse

The content in this appendix is not current and is of historical significance only.

who has completed a graduate degree nursing and has direct or indirect clinical practice involving clients with biopsychosocial alterations because of nervous system dysfunction. Specific neuroscience APN activities may be influenced by workforce fluctuations, development of related healthcare specialties, geographic and economic disparities, economic incentives, and consumer demand.

Expert clinical practice is the hallmark of advanced practice nursing. Clinical practice involves assessment, diagnosis, and management of client problems as well as health promotion. Primary generic responsibilities, regardless of specialty, identify the following responsibilities of the APN (American Association of Colleges of Nursing, 1998; American Nurses Association [ANA], 1996):

1. Plans and coordinates interventions from a multidisciplinary perspective.
2. Functions across the healthcare system and works with diverse populations.
3. Initiates and facilitates quality improvement initiatives.
4. Facilitates, conducts, and promotes utilization of research activities in practice.
5. Develops education strategies and evaluates effectiveness of educational interventions.
6. Recommends and influences social and healthcare policies.
7. Provides consultation to improve care.
8. Applies legal and ethical standards to complex situations.

Each of these responsibilities may be directly applied into specialty practice by the neuroscience APN (Villanueva et al., 2008). Interventions may occur from a collaborative or independent decision-making position.

Advanced Practice Roles in Neuroscience Nursing

A regulatory model for advanced practice nursing has been proposed (APRN Consensus Work Group & the National Council of State Boards of Nursing APRN Advisory Committee, 2008). Four advanced practice roles are designated: certified nurse midwife, certified nurse anesthetist, clinical nurse specialist, and nurse practitioner. This document focuses on the advanced practice roles found in neuroscience nursing.

Clinical Nurse Specialist (CNS)

The definition of a CNS is as follows: a registered nurse who is prepared at the master's or doctoral level and provides an advanced level of care in a specialized

area of nursing (ANA, 1976, 1980). Graduate-level education prepares the CNS to think critically and abstractly to assess care situations at an advanced level and to integrate research into clinical practice (National Council of State Boards of Nursing, 2002). Certification is required for licensure in many states; certification examinations are provided by the American Nurses Credentialing Center (ANCC) and the American Association of Critical Care Nurses. CNS practice is focused on three spheres of influence: the patient, nurse, and system and encompasses seven competencies: direct clinical practice, expert coaching and guidance, consultation, research, clinical and professional leadership, collaboration, and ethical decision making (National Association of Clinical Nurse Specialists, 2003, 2004).

The neuroscience CNS is typically centered in acute care. As an APN, the CNS role in direct clinical practice is focused on a patient or patient populations with complex needs. For example, the CNS may augment the care of a patient with increasing intracranial pressure using advanced assessment skills to plan emergent interventions to improve the patient's outcome and the nurses' skills via role modeling and mentorship. In addition, the CNS is directly involved with neuroscience patients at the population level such as the populations of traumatic brain injury or stroke patients. In this context, the CNS will review evidence-based literature and lead a multidisciplinary team in the development and implementation of treatment protocols that span the continuum of care: prehospital response, emergency department, intensive care unit, step-down unit, and rehabilitation. The CNS will analyze data on an ongoing basis to guide performance improvement initiatives to optimize patient outcomes. In this process, the CNS may also identify opportunities to conduct research to address clinical problems.

Nurse Practitioner (NP)

The definition of an NP is as follows: a registered nurse who is prepared, through advanced education and clinical training, to provide a wide range of preventative and acute healthcare services to individuals of all ages (American College of Nurse Practitioners, 2008a). Certification is required for licensure following completion of the program of study. National certification examinations are provided by the ANCC, the Academy of Nurse Practitioners, and the American Association of Critical Care Nurses. Currently, no NP programs have a dedicated program of study for neuroscience. NPs practicing in neuroscience have completed a program of study (e.g., adult health or acute care) and then directly practice with individuals with neuroscience disorders.

The content in this appendix is not current and is of historical significance only.

The role of the NP in the care of neuroscience patients is highly variable. Typical activities for a neuroscience NP may include performing a health history and examination (minor to comprehensive); ordering and interpreting appropriate laboratory tests and diagnostic studies; diagnosing and treating illness; promoting wellness and prevention of disease and injury; providing patient education and counseling; performing procedures; engaging in research, education, patient advocacy, and administrative duties; exercising autonomy in clinical decision making; working collaboratively with other members of the healthcare team; and providing these services in a cost-effective manner (American College of Nurse Practitioners, 2008b).

It is important to note that the CNS and NP roles may be blended in some settings, without distinct differences in work activities or responsibilities between the two titles (Klein, 2007). Both CNS and NP APNs may perform procedures, bill for services provided, and prescribe medications. Further, many nurses with CNS credentialing have undergone training in the NP role as well.

Environment for Neuroscience Advanced Practice Nursing

The neuroscience APN may be employed in any area where clients with biopsychosocial alterations because of nervous system dysfunction may be encountered. There are multiple practice sites for neuroscience patients such as hospitals, outpatient settings, private practice, academic institutions, research facilities, rehabilitation centers, and community settings. Client care may have a specific disease focus, such as neuro-oncology, specialty focus, such as neurosurgery, or problem focus, such as chronic pain management. Client care may be provided across the lifespan or within a specific age group (children or older adults). The role of the APN in a neuroscience practice may be specific or include many parts of the various groups and settings described. The following are examples of advanced practice applications but are by no means limited to these settings.

The APN may practice in the neurosurgery intensive care unit, providing direct patient care while mentoring staff nurses and orienting new graduates. Another APN may have pediatric neurosurgery as the specialty, performing preoperative and postoperative assessments of children and/or providing direct and indirect care to children in the intensive care unit with complex neurosurgical needs (e.g., traumatic brain injury, craniotomy for tumor resection, cranial vault remodeling, and neonates with myelomeningocele). Another APN may practice in the clinic setting, providing specialized care to elderly patients with movement disorders such as Parkinson's disease or myasthenia gravis or manage care for both inpatients and outpatients.

Another APN may work with a neuro-oncology team, coordinating radiation, chemotherapy, and surgical interventions all the while helping the patient navigate hospital bureaucracy. The APN working in the perioperative area conducts assessments, writes orders, and assists the neurosurgical team.

Education and Certification for Neuroscience APNs

The neuroscience APN has a specialized body of knowledge and expanded clinical skills acquired at the graduate level, with the master's degree as the minimum requirement for entry into advanced practice (American Association of Colleges of Nursing, 1998). The American Association of Neuroscience Nurses supports the concept of doctoral preparation for advanced practice nursing. Advanced practice certification via examination through the appropriate nationally recognized organization is a requirement for licensure. The ANCC offers nine certification examinations for NPs and nine certification examinations for CNSs in addition to four other advanced practice examinations (ANCC, 2008). Specialty nursing certifications examinations for advanced practice, such as those offered through the Oncology Nursing Certification Corporation, the Pediatric Nursing Credentialing Board, and the American Association of Critical Care Nurses Certification Corporation, may also be accepted for licensure.

Regulation of Advanced Practice

The nurse practice act and regulations promulgated by individual state boards of nursing delineate the scope of practice for the all APNs and the neuroscience APN in particular. Not all states currently recognize the CNS as an APN. In 23 states, NPs are allowed to practice independently without any physician involvement or supervision. Four states require physician involvement but do not require written documentation of that relationship. Twenty-four states still mandate physician supervision with documentation of this relationship (Pearson, 2008). APNs are required to hold at least two licenses to practice, one to practice as a registered nurse and the second to practice at the advanced level.

Institutions or practice groups may also require a collaborative practice agreement. The collaborative practice agreement delegates authority to the neuroscience APN and sets forth responsibilities mutually agreed upon by both the collaborating physician and the neuroscience APN. The agreement consists of (a) guidelines or protocols, (b) responsibilities, (c) evaluation, and (d) periodic reviews of protocols or guidelines. It also outlines direct, indirect, or remote levels of supervision required, which may be specific

The content in this appendix is not current and is of historical significance only.

for certain situations, and sets forth the manner in which the neuroscience APN will communicate with the collaborating physician, especially when the APN encounters a situation outside the scope of practice. Responsibilities might include procedures such as shunt taps, lumbar punctures, insertion of an intracranial monitor, application of spinal traction, or programming of a neurological device such as a shunt valve, deep brain stimulator, or intrathecal pump. Although all states provide some aspect of prescriptive authority to APNs, there is variability to the independence allowed (O'Malley & Mains, 2003). When permitted, prescriptive authority requires advanced pharmacology knowledge and compliance with state requirements for a particular specialty area. A collaborative practice agreement also serves to delineate prescriptive authority.

Summary

The neuroscience APN is challenged to provide care to patients and families within a complex and constantly changing healthcare environment. The role of the neuroscience APN is multifaceted and variable. It is crucial for the neuroscience APN to be aware of the diverse statutes governing their practice and practice within their defined scope of practice. This document serves to assist the neuroscience APN in developing a framework for practice.

Neuroscience Advanced Practice Nurse Standards of Practice

Standard I. Assessment

The neuroscience advanced practice nurse collects comprehensive data to make clinical decisions and positively impact patient outcomes for the patient with neurological dysfunction.

Measurement Criteria
The neuroscience advanced practice nurse:

1. Systematically conducts a comprehensive examination, based on health history, age, cultural background, patient complaint, and potential causes of neurological dysfunction.

   a. Utilizes all available sources of information, including family members, caregivers, other interdisciplinary healthcare team members, healthcare records, and system data as relevant.

   b. Utilizes appropriate assessment techniques, incorporating technological data and diagnostic information where appropriate.

2. Initiates and interprets diagnostic tests and procedures as permitted by state nurse practice act or credentialing body.

3. Prioritizes data collection based on patient condition, anticipated needs, or environmental situation.
4. Identifies family or caregiver needs that influence patient outcomes.
5. Identifies system and personnel needs in the clinical environment that influence patient outcomes.
6. Synthesizes data to identify patient risks and needs, refocusing data collection and prioritization on an ongoing basis.
7. Documents relevant assessment data in a confidential, accessible, and retrievable format.

Standard II. Diagnosis

The neuroscience advance practice nurse uses information obtained from assessment data to formulate diagnoses for the patient with neurological dysfunction.

Measurement Criteria
The neuroscience advanced practice nurse:

1. Collaboratively develops and prioritizes diagnoses, consulting other members of the interdisciplinary healthcare team as necessary.

   a. Systematically compares and contrasts findings to determine differential diagnoses where appropriate.

2. Validates diagnoses with the patient, family, and other interdisciplinary healthcare team members to improve communication and adherence to the treatment plan, revising diagnoses as necessary.
3. Documents diagnoses in a manner that facilitates communication among the interdisciplinary team and determination of expected outcomes and plan of care.

Standard III. Outcome Identification

The neuroscience advance practice nurse develops individualized, diagnosis-based expected outcomes for the patient with neurological dysfunction.

Measurement Criteria
The neuroscience advanced practice nurse:

1. Derives outcomes from assessment and diagnostic data that include time frames and provide direction for care.
2. Establishes outcomes to measure effectiveness of interventions, modifying outcomes in response to changing needs or condition.
3. Mutually formulates outcomes with the patient, family, and interdisciplinary healthcare team members.
4. Formulates developmentally and culturally appropriate, cost-effective, and realistic outcomes in relation to capabilities and available resources.

The content in this appendix is not current and is of historical significance only.

5. Identifies outcomes that are consistent with clinical practice and current scientific evidence and are ethically sound.
6. Analyzes factors that hinder achievement of outcomes for patients, families, nurses, or systems.
7. Documents outcomes in a manner that facilitates outcome measurement and communication among the interdisciplinary team.

Standard IV. Planning

The neuroscience advance practice nurse develops a comprehensive plan of care to achieve expected outcomes for the patient with neurological dysfunction.

Measurement Criteria
The neuroscience advanced practice nurse:

1. Develops a mutually derived plan of care with the patient, using assessment data, evidence-based practice interventions, and theoretical knowledge.

   a. Includes the patient and family needs, values, beliefs, and resources in developing the plan of care.
   b. Considers cost, benefits, and alternatives in developing the plan of care.
   c. Addresses disease prevention, health promotion, and health maintenance in the plan of care.

2. Creates, advises, and influences system-level policies that affect programs of care.
3. Documents the plan of care outcomes in a manner that facilitates implementation of the plan and communication among the interdisciplinary team.

Standard V. Implementation

The neuroscience advance practice nurse implements the plan of care to achieve expected outcomes for the patient with neurological dysfunction.

Measurement Criteria
The neuroscience advanced practice nurse:

1. Reviews the set of all possible interventions and possible consequences associated with each intervention.

   a. Considers available resources, costs, risks, and benefits for each intervention.
   b. Assures interventions are ethical, developmentally and culturally appropriate, and based on best available evidence.

2. Recommends, selects, and/or orders interventions as permitted by state nurse practice act or credentialing body.

   a. Establishes algorithms, standing orders, or practice guidelines.

b. Prescribes pharmacological and nonpharmacological interventions according to patient needs, best available evidence, and physiologic principles.
c. Monitors responses to interventions with specific attention to potential adverse effects.
d. Adjusts interventions on an ongoing basis as needed.
e. Provides the patient with information about interventions, including intended effects, potential risks, possible alternatives, costs, and patient role.

3. Performs interventions in a safe and ethical manner or delegates interventions where appropriate.
4. Assures coordination of care and patient and family involvement to meet individualized needs.

   a. Provides consultation based on defined role responsibilities.
   b. Provides referrals based on cost and benefit considerations.
   c. Implements recommendations from referral sources as appropriate.

5. Initiates and sustains collaborative relationships among healthcare teams to facilitate interdisciplinary interventions.
6. Incorporates system and community resources when implementing interventions.
7. Documents responses to interventions implemented in a manner that demonstrates accountability, minimizes error, and facilitates communication among the interdisciplinary team and outcome measurement.

Standard VI. Evaluation

The neuroscience advance practice nurse evaluates progress in attainment of expected outcomes for the patient with neurological dysfunction.

Measurement Criteria
The neuroscience advanced practice nurse:

1. Conducts a systematic, ongoing evaluation of expected outcomes.

   a. Includes the patient, family, other interdisciplinary healthcare team members, and system in the evaluation process.
   b. Incorporates advanced nursing knowledge, quality scientific indicators, and best available evidence into evaluative measures.

2. Analyzes findings from evaluative measures to assess effectiveness of the plan in attaining outcomes.
3. Revises the diagnoses, expected outcomes, plan of care, and interventions to address outcomes that have not been met or have been only partially met.
4. Disseminates evaluation findings to the patient family, other interdisciplinary healthcare team

The content in this appendix is not current and is of historical significance only.

members, and system to improve overall quality, satisfaction, and safety of care.

5. Documents the evaluation performed and any necessary revisions to the diagnoses, expected outcomes, plan of care, or interventions.

Neuroscience Advanced Practice Nurse Standards of Professional Performance
Standard I. Quality of Care

The neuroscience advanced practice nurse systematically evaluates the quality and effectiveness of nursing practice.

Measurement Criteria
The neuroscience advanced practice nurse:

1. Uses current evidenced-based treatment interventions to promote optimal patient outcomes while maintaining patient safety and considering cost.
2. Participates in quality of care activities as appropriate to the individual's education, experience, and position.

   a. Systematically develops criteria for evaluating the quality and effectiveness of nursing practice as well as organizational systems to assess quality of care.
   b. Collects and analyzes data to monitor quality care and uses these data to formulate recommendations to improve nursing practice and patient outcomes.

3. Assumes a leadership role in the development of policies, procedures, and practice guidelines to improve quality of care and patient outcomes as a clinical expert.
4. Utilizes an interdisciplinary approach to assure quality, evidence-based, cost-effective holistic care for the neuroscience patient.

Standard II. Performance Appraisal

The neuroscience advanced practice nurse continuously evaluates one's own practice in relation to professional practice standards and relevant statutes and regulations and is accountable to the public and profession for providing competent clinical care.

Measurement Criteria
The neuroscience advanced practice nurse:

1. Demonstrates knowledge of current professional practice standards, laws, and regulations through practice.
2. Engages in performance appraisal on a regular basis, seeking constructive feedback regarding one's

own practice according to professional standards and identifying areas of strength and areas where professional development would be beneficial.

3. Incorporates role performance reviews from peers, professional colleagues, clients, and others as appropriate into practice.

Standard III. Education

The neuroscience advanced practice nurse acquires and maintains current knowledge and competency in advanced nursing practice.

Measurement Criteria
The neuroscience advanced practice nurse:

1. Participates in ongoing educational activities related to clinical and theoretical knowledge and professional issues.
2. Seeks experiences to acquire and maintain clinical skills and competence appropriate to area of practice.
3. Maintains professional certification and obtains continuing education as required for licensure.

Standard IV. Collegiality

The neuroscience advanced practice nurse contributes to the professional development of nursing and other healthcare colleagues.

The neuroscience advanced practice nurse:

1. Shares knowledge and skills with colleagues and members of the multidisciplinary team and models expert practice.
2. Promotes a healthy work environment that is conducive to safe and effective patient care.
3. Partners with others to promote an environment conducive to the clinical education of students, nurses, and healthcare team members.
4. Interacts with colleagues on both a local and national level to enhance one's own professional nursing practice.
5. Participates in professional organizations to improve the quality of nursing care and optimize patient outcomes.

Standard V. Ethics

The neuroscience advanced practice nurse formulates decisions on patient care and acts on behalf of the patient with neurological dysfunction by using ethical principles and systematic criteria.

Measurement Criteria
The neuroscience advanced practice nurse:

1. Utilizes the *Code of Ethics for Nurses With Interpretive Statements* to guide practice.

The content in this appendix is not current and is of historical significance only.

2. Provides nondiscriminatory care to diverse populations while maintaining patient confidentiality within legal and regulatory parameters.
3. Acts as a patient advocate while maintaining a therapeutic and professional relationship with the patient.
4. Informs the patient of expected healthcare outcomes including anticipated risks, potential benefits, and possible alternatives while supporting care that preserves patient autonomy, dignity and rights.
5. Contributes to the resolution of ethical dilemmas of both systems and individuals through an interdisciplinary approach.

Standard VI. Collaboration

The neuroscience advanced practice nurse collaborates with patients, families, nurses, physicians, other healthcare providers, and relevant system parties when assessing, planning, delivering, and evaluating the care of a patient or group of patients with neurological dysfunction.

Measurement Criteria

The neuroscience advanced practice nurse:

1. Collaborates with the patient, family, nurse, and other healthcare providers in the formulation of overall goals and the plan of care and in decisions related to care and the delivery of services.
2. Facilitates the formation of an interdisciplinary team to work collaboratively to optimize patient outcomes.
3. Serves as a mentor to nurses and other healthcare team members.
4. Consults with and makes referrals to appropriate providers to ensure that the full spectrum of the patient needs is met across the continuum of care.

Standard VII. Research

The neuroscience advance practice nurse integrates research into practice.

Measurement Criteria

The neuroscience advance practice nurse:

1. Utilizes the best available evidence to guide practice interventions and advance patient care.

   a. Critically appraises research for practice application.
   b. Critically appraises practice in the context of best available evidence.

2. Utilizes research to enhance the environment of care and improve patient outcomes.

   a. Utilizes research skills in problem evaluation.

3. Participates in research activities appropriate to education, experience, and environment. Activities may include the following:

   a. Identifies and prioritizes research problems of concern to neuroscience nursing.
   b. Participates in data collection.
   c. Participates in a research program at the organizational level.
   d. Disseminates research findings through all available avenues.
   e. Conducts research to advance patient care.
   f. Encourages and facilitates the neuroscience nursing research agenda.
   g. Utilizes research findings to develop clinical guidelines, policies, and procedures.

Standard VIII. Resource Utilization

The neuroscience advance practice nurse considers factors related to safety, efficacy, and fiscal responsibility when delivering care for the patient with neurological dysfunction.

Measurement Criteria

The neuroscience advance practice nurse:

1. Integrates safety, efficacy, and cost considerations into practice decisions as part of an interdisciplinary approach to care.
2. Facilitates patient and family access to appropriate care resources.
3. Delegates tasks based upon patient condition, skills of the designated caregiver, potential for harm, complexity of the task, and predictability of the outcome.
4. Serves as a resource to influence healthcare policy.
5. Advocates for patient rights, an optimal care environment, access to care, and improved quality of care.
6. Develops innovations to maximize safety, efficacy, and cost-effectiveness of care.

References

American Association of Colleges of Nursing. (1998). *Certification and regulation of advanced practice nurse (AACN position statement)*. Retrieved December 15, 2008, from www.aacn.nche.edu/Publications/positions/cereg.htm

American College of Nurse Practitioners. (2008a). *What is a nurse practitioner?* Retrieved December 15, 2008, from www.acpnweb.org/i4a/pages/index.cfm?pageid+3479

American College of Nurse Practitioners. (2008b). *Numbers of nurse practitioners*. Retrieved December 15, 2008, from www.acpnweb.org/i4a/pages/index.cfm?pageid=3353

American Nurses Association. (1976). *Description of practice: Clinical nurse specialist in the scope of nursing practice*. Kansas City, MO: Author.

The content in this appendix is not current and is of historical significance only.

American Nurses Association. (1980). *Nursing: A social policy statement.* Kansas City, MO: Author.

American Nurses Association. (1996). *Scope and standards of advanced practice registered nursing.* Washington, DC: Author.

American Nurses Credentialing Center. (2008). *Certification.* Retrieved December 15, 2008, from http://www.nursecredentialing.org/certification.aspx

APRN Consensus Work Group & the National Council of State Boards of Nursing APRN Advisory Committee. (2008). *Consensus model for APRN regulation: Licensure, accreditation, certification, & education.* Retrieved July 16, 2009, from http://www.bne.state.tx.us/practice/pdfs/aprnmodel.pdf

Herrmann, L., & Zabramski, J. M. (2005). Tandem practice model: A model for physician–nurse practitioner collaboration in a specialty practice, neurosurgery. *Journal of the Academy of Nurse Practitioners, 17*(6), 213–218.

Klein, T. A. (2007). Scope of practice and the nurse practitioner: Regulation, competency, expansion, and evolution. *Topics in Advanced Practice Nursing, 7*(3). Retrieved December 15, 2008, from www.medscape.com/viewprogram/4188.pnt

National Association of Clinical Nurse Specialists. (2003). Regulatory credentialing of clinical nurse specialists. *Clinical Nurse Specialist, 17*(3), 163–169.

National Association of Clinical Nurse Specialists. (2004). *Statement on clinical nurse specialist practice and education.* Harrisburg, PA: Author.

National Council of State Boards of Nursing. (2002). *Position paper: Regulation of advanced practice nursing.* Retrieved December 15, 2008, from www.ncsbn.org/public/regulations/res/APRN_Position_Paper2002.pdf

O'Malley, P., & Mains, J. (2003). Update on prescriptive authority for the clinical nurse specialist. *Clinical Nurse Specialist, 17*(4), 191–193.

Pearson, L. (2008). The Pearson report. *American Journal for Nurse Practitioners, 12*(2), 9–80.

Villanueva, N., Blank-Reid, C., Stewart-Amidei, C., Cartwright, C., Haymore, J., & Jones, R. (2008). The role of the advanced practice nurse in neuroscience nursing: Results of the 2006 AANN membership survey. *Journal of Neuroscience Nursing, 40*(2), 119–124.

Webb, D. (2000). Scope of neuroscience nursing. In C. Stewart-Amidei & J.A. Kunkel (Eds.), *AANN's neuroscience nursing: Human responses to neurologic dysfunction* (2nd ed., pp. 3–11). Philadelphia: Saunders.

Index

Note: Entries with [2002] and [2010] indicate an entry from *Scope and Standards of Neuroscience Nursing Practice (2002)*, reproduced in Appendix A, and *Scope and Standards of Practice for Neuroscience Advanced Practice Nurses (2010)*, reproduced in Appendix B respectively. That information is not current but included for historical value only.